CANCER KICKIN'
WARRIOR

CANCER KICKIN'
WARRIOR

The ultimate feel-good cancer survivor book

Richard,
We are warriors
and living proof that
life is great and worth
fighting for. Live it to the fullest.
Best Wishes,
J.W.
10/26/10

INEZ WHITEHEAD-DICKENS

Illustrations by David Tate and Marshall Sampson

authorHOUSE®

AuthorHouse™
1663 Liberty Drive
Bloomington, IN 47403
www.authorhouse.com
Phone: 1-800-839-8640

First published by AuthorHouse 9/23/2010

ISBN: 978-1-4520-5505-3 (e)
ISBN: 978-1-4520-5504-6 (sc)
ISBN: 978-1-4520-5503-9 (hc)

Library of Congress Control Number: 2010913864

Printed in the United States of America

This book is printed on acid-free paper.

I dedicate this book to my beautiful grandchildren, Mekhi, Kain, Kailynn, and my cousins Gary, Clara, D. Channsin Berry, and family; Jack and Virdell; Kitty and Ronnie and my dear friends Bill and Renee Goodwin.

A special dedication to Charlene, the ultimate warrior!

This book was written in memory of
Dick Fenoff and Carmen Cors

David and Marion Whitehead and aunt Inez, rest in peace knowing you produced a strong, caring daughter and niece.

ACKNOWLEDGMENTS

When I first thought about writing this book, I came up with a million reasons why I couldn't. But people like my husband, Mike; my children, especially, Marshall, David, and Dre; my daughter-in-law, Amirh; and my dear friends Bootie (who kept kickin' me all the way), Joyce, Renee, Betty, Elba, Rose, Margaret, and others (there are too many to mention) kept encouraging me and expressed so much faith in me that I couldn't let them down.

I am eternally grateful to my fellow warriors whose stories appear in this book. Without them this book would not have been possible.

I want to thank the soldiers who continue to work tirelessly and give their love and support to all of the Cancer Kickin' Warriors. A special thanks to Susan Campriello, who is an award-winning reporter for *The Catskill Daily Mail*. In 2010 she took home the award for Distinguished Online Breaking News Coverage. Susan has been instrumental in bringing our cancer-fighting issues to the forefront. She has a heart the size of Texas and never fails to give all pertinent medical stories, and not just cancer, a voice. She has worked tirelessly with us in our quest to improve the rights of cancer patients.

Patty and Joyce, from the beginning you made it clear to me that dying was not an option.

Pat V., Cyndee, Betty, and Terry—every year, you walked with me.

WHY I WROTE THIS BOOK

When I was diagnosed with advanced breast cancer in 2001, I was frozen in time. At that time, the only thing I knew about any cancer, is that if you have it, you die. I agonized over things like, am I going to dwindle away and die a painful death? How do I tell my kids? Do I have enough time to get things in order? Who will take care of my husband? My mind went on and on. I looked for someone to talk to who had been diagnosed with my stage of cancer. When I couldn't find any, I thought the worst. I was told that once people go through their ordeal with cancer, they don't want to talk about it. I got on my knees and promised God that if he got me through this, I would become that voice.

Well he kept his end of the bargain, and I'm keeping mine. But the stories in this book are not just about me; they are about people who have fought and won their battles with every type and stage of cancer. In talking to them, I learned so much. The trauma one goes through from the beginning of the diagnosis to the end of the treatments makes it understandable that people want to forget it once it's over. But the people in this book wanted to share their stories to let anyone going through this to know it is not a death sentence, and more important—there is life after cancer! Belief in God, positive thinking, and a strong support system will see you through any trial.

The stories in this book are also about the people who stand with us and fight for us in the battle against cancer. Without them, we wouldn't survive.

So when you read these stories, look at not only the type of cancer they survived, but also the faith, love, and support they had. In some cases you will see how cancer changed their life for the better. So look at their lives post-cancer. Look at their strong, loving support system. When you feel depressed or feel like giving up, pick up this book and read one of the many inspirational stories. You'll learn not to be afraid of cancer; only be afraid if you don't do something about it. Then I guarantee, you too can become not just a survivor, but a *Cancer Kickin' Warrior!*

CHAPTER ONE

DISCOVERY

"Hi Inez, this is Dr. Alli. I have your results from your test and I would like you to come into the office Monday. Oh, and please bring Mike with you." Does this statement sound familiar, warriors? Needless to say I was nervous, because I had seen Dr. Alli numerous times before, and she had never commanded an appearance by my husband, Mike.

When we went into her office, she took us in immediately. I was surprised to see that there weren't any other patients in the office. She sat me down and held my hand. I said in my mind, *Uh-oh! This isn't good.* To be honest with you, I was prepared to hear the word *cancer*, but I wasn't prepared to hear, "Inez, your test shows you have breast cancer and it's pretty advanced. It appears to have spread outside your left breast and into your chest wall.

The reason I was totally taken off guard was because I had had a mammogram and an ultrasound of the breast in July 2000. Here we were, only eight months later, and I was being told I had advanced breast cancer. It was psychologically damaging to me because I was your typical type A—the one everyone goes to, a control freak—but I didn't know how I was going to control this.

At that time, the room got smaller and I felt like I was going to pass out. But then I looked at my husband, who was as white as a sheet, and somehow I was able to pull it together. Picture this: I had a doctor with tears in her eyes and a husband about to faint, and I was the one who had to hold them together. Go figure!

Even though the doctor's office was only a few miles from our house, it seemed like the drive home took forever. I can remember the ghostly calm that came over the car. Mike didn't say anything; I couldn't say anything. I just stared out the window in a total fog. When I arrived home, I went to my room, closed the door, and just cried. I was wondering just how long I had to live. You know, we all know we are not going to live forever, but damn, I didn't think forever would end so soon. I always felt like I was the glue that held everyone together, the go-getter, the strong one in the family. Now I felt like nothing.

In December 2000, I had been in the hospital for treatment of a lung infection. They had put me on steroids, so when I felt what appeared to be a raised muscle just above my breast, I thought it was the result of the steroids. When I came off the medication, the lump didn't go away. I was due to go back to the doctor and have my lungs checked because of the infection. While I was there, I showed the doctor the lump. At the time, she didn't feel it was anything, but she sent me for a mammogram.

Now, let me tell you, folks, because I had two benign lumps removed in 1989 and 1991, I was always faithful about getting my annual mammograms and ultrasounds of the breast.

I should have sensed something was wrong, because as I was putting my clothes back on, the technician came out and said, "Oh, Mrs. Dickens, we just want to get a few more pictures." Usually, I was in and out with these things, but not this time! I asked if there was anything wrong, and he assured me it was just routine. Yeah, right! The tech told me the doctor would get the results in a few days and call me. Well folks, let me tell you a few days turned into a few hours, because she called me that night to tell me not to worry; but she wanted to schedule me for a biopsy. When I asked if anything was wrong, she said the results of my other tests were inconclusive.

I went in and had a surgical biopsy. I was still groggy when I came out of the anesthesia, but I could have sworn I heard my surgeon talking to another doctor using the word *cancer*.

When I asked her if they were talking about me, she said no and that they wouldn't have my results for a few days. She told me to get some rest. So back I went to la-la land.

That night, I got that fateful call that introduced this whole story!

While we were in her office, the doctor explained that the cancer was in my left breast and had spread into my chest wall. The tests also picked up calcifications in my right breast. Dr. Alli went over my options. Before she could get through all of them, I interrupted her and said, "I want it out! I want surgery, chemo, and radiation—hit me with everything you've got." I also said I wanted both breasts removed, since they had picked up calcifications in the right breast. I wasn't going to go through getting a mammogram every six months and worrying if I had another occurrence of cancer. The stress would give me a heart attack.

When I mentioned the mastectomy, she turned to my husband and asked him how he felt about it. People, let me tell you, I immediately said, "Never mind what he thinks; this is my life, and this is what I want." My husband quickly concurred.

We agreed to have the mastectomy and implants done at the same time. If I had to do it again, I wouldn't recommend that. I'll tell you about that later. I had to consult with a cosmetic surgeon. When I explained the urgency of the situation, she said she could set it up for May, two months later! Hello, I have stage 3B breast cancer! I called my doctor crying and hysterical. She agreed to talk to the surgeon. A quick callback later, and they scheduled me for surgery the following week. About now, are you wondering why I just didn't go to another cosmetic surgeon? You have to remember, I was scared, and I didn't know zilch about cosmetic surgery or cancer. My doctor said this one was good, so I went with her.

The surgery itself went well. But when I awoke, the surgeon told me they couldn't get all of the cancer because it had spread to my chest wall, so the only other option was to try to kill it with radiation. On a good note, upon returning to my room, my good friend Pat, whom I hadn't seen in years and was also a breast cancer survivor, was there looking down on me and smiling.

Now mind you, I had a bilateral mastectomy. So you can imagine the physical and mental pain I was going through. Well, folks, this was right around the time the insurance companies had the bright idea to have basically a drive-through mastectomy. Can you imagine, the hospital was going to send me home the same day? I pitched a fit. I was hysterical. My husband, who is usually very laid-back, was on the phone with anyone who would listen. Needless to say, they kept me for four days. Thinking back, I jokingly say that they probably changed my claim from breast cancer to mental illness. Let that be a lesson to you all. As my old boss use to say, the squeaky wheel gets the oil.

The first couple of days I was at home, I had a visiting nurse to change my dressing on my wounds, but then my husband took over. I have to tell you the first time he unwrapped the dressing, I started to recoil, wondering how he would feel looking at nothing but a scarred area. Now mind you, I never was a voluptuous woman. Sensing my reaction, he said, "You know, if I was looking for a woman with big ones, do you really think I would have married you?"

This made me laugh and put me at ease. I think at this time he felt proud to be able to do something to help me through this horrific time in my life. I sometimes believe that cancer is harder on the family, because they feel so helpless. Right now, you may be wondering where my kids fit in to all of this. That I will get to in a little bit.

CHAPTER TWO

TREATMENT

Next, the surgeon referred me to an oncologist who was suppose to be tops in his field. Well, at my one and only visit with him, I was asking him questions, and the response was always with a sigh and a terse, "Yes, Inez?" I went back to my doctor and demanded another oncologist. She said I didn't understand that the one she had recommended was number one in his field. I said, "Well, then give me number two, because if I'm going to die, it isn't going to be in this guy's hands."

So I went to the oncologist whom I am still seeing to this day—Dr. Patrick DiPaolo. I am a very direct person. All I knew about cancer at the time was that it kills you. So at my first visit, I simply asked him when I was going to die, because I had four kids at home and I had to prepare them. He bowed his head and then looked up and said, "Well, you know it's metastasized, so the only thing I can say is, if you do what I say, I can only guarantee you'll live to be ninety. After that, I can't promise you anything!" He further stated, "Who knows when they are going to die?" Folks, I can't tell you the boost this gave me. Here I went into his office talking about death, and he sent me out talking about life. People, believe me when I say that attitude and the right doctor make all the difference in the world as far as recovery goes.

He explained to me that I was going to receive eight rounds of chemotherapy followed by six weeks of daily radiation. The chemotherapy would consist of four weeks of a cocktail mixture of cyclophosphamide and Adriamycin followed by four weeks of Taxol. In order to endure the chemotherapy, I was going to have a portacath implanted right above my breast. This was a device surgically put in that administered IV medicine directly into the vein. So I scheduled a time to have that surgically implanted.

Well, about three days after the port was inserted, I went back to the doctor for a checkup. Mike and I had planned to go to a movie and dinner after the visit. The doctor was checking my lungs and asked me if I was having trouble breathing. Being asthmatic, I told her I was always short of breath. She told me she wanted me to go straight to the emergency room for a chest x-ray. I explained that we were on our way to a "date" and that I would go the next week. She insisted I go right then and there and called the hospital to inform them that I was coming.

We reluctantly went to the hospital and had the chest x-ray. I got dressed and was literally walking out the door, when a physician ran up to me and asked where I was going. I said, "To a movie and dinner."

He said, "Mrs. Dickens, your right lung has 100% collapse; you are not going anywhere. We have a thoracic surgeon en route as we speak!"

I started yelling, "Mike, tell them they're wrong. I'm fine," as they whisked me into a side room. Mike tried to argue, but they showed him the x-ray and explained the urgency of the situation. Within minutes, a doctor came in with a nurse, introduced himself, and explained the procedure. And *wham*, with no anesthesia, he stuck a tube in my side to inflate my lung. It felt like someone had stabbed me. They were amazed I was able to walk with my lung collapsed.

During my healing process from this, I noticed that one of my implants was getting smaller. When I went back to the surgeon after a month, I mentioned this to her. She ordered an MRI, and as luck would have it, one of my boobies was deflating! Now, I don't know whether the port punctured it or it was a manufacture defect. They didn't want to operate to remove it, because I was scheduled for chemotherapy. One of the many side effects of chemotherapy is that you're subject to infections. So I had to persevere with one young, perky booby and one old, saggy-looking one!

Now, Dr. DiPaolo told me that with the type of chemotherapy regimen I was going to endure, I would more than likely lose my hair. When I discussed this with my hubby, Mike—who, by the way, was slowly going bald himself—he suggested we shave my head so that I wouldn't have to go through the trauma of seeing my hair fall out. So Mike shaved my head, and as we stood side by side looking in the mirror, he affectionately said, "See, now we look like twins." People, I can't tell you what it does to the healing process to have such strong love and support from your mate.

My first session with chemo didn't go too badly. But by the second, I started feeling sick after the treatment. By the third, I was feeling weaker and throwing up a lot. But the craziest thing happened: I had cravings for strawberry milk shakes and fried chicken. I thought, *if I'm pregnant, I'm selling my story to the* Enquirer! I told this to the doctor, who got a laugh out of it. He explained that if that was the only thing I could hold down, go for it, but don't eat a bucket at a time. Mike brought a juicer, and I learned to love the veggie drinks. He became a master of the mixer.

You know, chemotherapy can be rough for some people, but I know a friend of mine who went to work right after treatment. Unfortunately, that wasn't me! There were times when Mike had to literally hold me up to walk to the car after a treatment. I looked like I was drunk. There were times when I would feel so sick and weak, I was wondering if I was really dying and no one had the courage to tell me. But I kept fighting. At this time, I also experienced what has come to be known as "chemo brain." That is when you go through a period of forgetfulness. I thought it was Alzheimer's, but I was assured this was normal and would pass. Now, nine years later, if I forget something, I blame it on chemo brain.

Right at the end of my chemo treatments, I woke up feeling like my right breast was on fire. This was the one that had deflated. Mike took me to the hospital. I had a fever of 103°, and my blood count had dropped to transfusion level. Due to the cancer, they didn't want to immediately perform a transfusion, so they tried to nutritionally bring my blood count up. They admitted me to the hospital, and for the next week I lived on antibiotics, nutrients, and hospital food—which wasn't bad! They removed the implant and implanted another one in its place.

Would you believe, I noticed the left one was getting hard and extremely painful. After a trip back to a breast surgeon and more tests, it was determined I had capsular contracture. This is a common side affect with breast implants, because you are placing a foreign object into your body and its initial reaction is to reject it. So back to surgery I went, getting a replacement on the other side. As I stated before, I was never a well-endowed woman in that area, so I think every time an implant was put in, my body was rebelling, saying, *what the heck are these things?* I developed another infection, and for six weeks I walked around with a shunt in my arm and went daily for IV antibiotic treatment.

As you probably have gathered by now, I am a fighter and usually a very upbeat person. But after this, I was slowly sinking into depression. But one day while I was home watching TV, recovering from this surgery, they interrupted my program to say that one of the Twin Towers had been hit. As I watched this horrific story unfolding week after week, they started talking about the people who had lost their lives in the 9/11 attack. All who succumbed on 9/11 left their house that morning not knowing they would never return. It was then I had an epiphany. I said to myself, *here were people younger than me and probably healthier than me, and in a flash their life was over. They never even had a chance to say good-bye to their loved ones.* So why the hell was I feeling sorry for myself? Having cancer meant I just had something with a name. It didn't mean I was going to live longer, but it also didn't mean my time was going to be shorter on this earth. The people who succumbed on 9/11 didn't know what they were fighting; but I did! I always say, if you know what you are fighting, you have a better chance of winning.

So I completed my chemotherapy sessions and made preparations for radiation. I went through several tests. One picked up cysts on my liver, but the radiologist didn't seem concerned. I went to radiation daily, Monday through Friday, for six weeks.

The radiation went fairly well. My only complaint was the extreme fatigue, which is par for the course.

All went well until December 2006, I was watching TV, and I felt a burning sensation in my left breast. As the day went on, the pain became more intense. I had to call Mike at work to ask him to come home. We immediately went to my primary doctor, Dr. Scott, who thought it was an infection. He sent me for an MRI, and sure enough, it was an infection—a *bad* infection. He called around to find a surgeon to look at it. He finally found one, and I was told to go to the hospital immediately.

It was there I met Dr. Berman, one of the most caring, compassionate doctors that I know. He explained that he was going to admit me and put me on a twenty-four-hour IV antibiotic treatment. If the infection did not improve, he would have to operate. Of course, the latter occurred. So out went another implant, and trust me, folks; this time it stayed out!

In 2007, on a visit to my primary doctor, she noticed a swelling in my neck. She wanted me to see an endocrinologist. I immediately thought, *Oh no, not again!* I thank Dr. McKeon for being such a thorough doctor. If she sees something out of whack, she jumps on it. The endocrinologist gave me tests, including an ultrasound. It came back as undetermined, so he suggested we wait six months to see if it changed. Six months later, I had another ultrasound done, and the cyst had grown. They still couldn't determine whether or not it was cancerous, so we decided to remove my left thyroid. Remember, people, cancer is not something you play around with. If something is getting bigger, your body is trying to tell you something. Luckily, I didn't need any follow-up medication. I have it checked every two years.

CHAPTER THREE

TELLING THE KIDS

When I first learned I had breast cancer, I was in shock. Then to find out I was in such an advanced stage … well, I was devastated. Like any good mother, I first wondered how I was going to tell my kids. I had four kids, three boys and one girl, ranging in age from twenty-three to thirty-one. Two of the boys David and Marshall, were still living at home, and even though they were adults, they still were mama's boys—though they would never admit it.

Mike and I discussed my options. I decided that, even though I was in an advanced stage of cancer, I would just tell them I had cancer. The word *cancer* in itself is scary enough as it is. I decided to wait and see how the treatments went. If I found I was getting progressively worse, then

I would tell them the whole story. You see, when I was a single parent, my kids saw me survive many struggles. They thought I walked on water, except when Marshall had to hold me up when I was studying math for college. Marshall became the parent, sitting up night after night with me, pounding a formula in my head; but that's another story. Mike and I were worried enough for everyone. As it turned out, that was the best decision I ever made in my life. I would advise anyone diagnosed with cancer, to not unload everything at one time on your children. The cancer patient's mind and time are completely occupied by the whirlwind of treatments, procedures, and doctor visits. But anyone sitting on the sidelines feels totally helpless and scared. So the day I told them, it went like this: "Listen, kids, I had a test done and it came back positive for breast cancer. Your dad and I have consulted a doctor and surgeon, and we decided the best treatment is to have a bilateral mastectomy." Now, as I was saying this, I noticed my youngest son Marshall's, eyes welling up with tears. So I gathered every bit of strength I could muster and said, "Now, why are you getting so upset? This is no big deal; you're making me scared." This seemed to calm the waters for a while. The only thing that troubled me was that Marshall worked for the same company I worked for, so he constantly had people coming up to him asking how I was. Sometimes they wanted graphic details. Some meant well; some were just nosy. So it was constantly on his mind. Mandy and Joe internalized it more, but living in another state removed them from the immediate situation.

I made it a point to never shed a tear around my kids. I saved my crying time for when they were at work. If I was extremely sick after a chemo session, I would always be "asleep" when they came home. I made every effort to put on a little lip gloss and greet them with a happy, upbeat attitude. The only one I allowed myself to show any emotions to was my faithful dog, Chloe, who appeared to understand everything.

I ran my sons and husband ragged, running to the store picking up my milk shakes and fried chicken to satisfy my cravings. When I became bald as a billiard ball, my sons told me they really liked my new look. Yeah, right! They took turns taking me to my treatments. My son David must have felt like he was "driving Ms. Daisy"!

David, along with Mike, took turns doing the cooking, cleaning, laundry, and chauffeuring. I have to say, they really pampered me, which made me feel like a princess in spite of what I was facing. They encouraged me, even yelled at me, when I had moments of feeling sorry for myself. David shamed me into getting into the driver's seat of the car, the first time since my diagnosis.

Another friend of the family whom I "adopted" is Andre. He can't do enough for me and my family. He is a part of us, whom I love dearly. At every family function, Andre's there.

In addition, I have three stepchildren: Shanell, Westley, and Felicia. I also have a beautiful daughter-in-law, Amirh, and four grandchildren I simply adore: Mekhi, Kain, Kailynn, and little Westley.

CHAPTER FOUR

MY LIFE BEFORE

Let me tell you a little about myself before I met Mr. Breast Cancer. That's right; I decided to give it a masculine tagline, because look what women go through: MENopause, MENstruation…You get the picture. Anyway, I was divorced, raising four kids. We used to spend a lot of time together, going to Keansburg Amusement Park, the beach, and carnivals. During this time, I met my husband, Mike, who was going through a divorce and had three children: Westley, Shanell, and Felicia. Now, prior to this, I was done with the dating scene. I had told my mother that I was through with men, and the only way I was going to meet one was if God dropped him on my doorstep. She said, "Toots"—that was her nickname for me—"if it's meant to be, it will be." Well,

Mike was painting houses on the side, and my father hired him to paint my house. And the rest is history. So, I guess you can say that God dropped him on my doorstep. We joined the two families together and became the Dickens bunch. We would pack the kids into the van and head off to wherever. The kids blended well. They quickly referred to each other as brother or sister.

I was working as a service representative for New Jersey Bell Telephone Company ...which turned into Bell Atlantic ... which turned into Verizon. I started off as the worst seller in the state. At the time, my attitude was, *I was hired to be a service representative, not a seller.* But my much-loved manager at the time, Doris, told me that New Jersey Bell was going to eventually be going into sales, and it was going to be an integral part of my job. I was still stubborn. My sales techniques went something like this: "Sir, you don't want call waiting, do you?" Well, needless to say, that didn't go over too well. Again, Doris gave me her *strong* pep talk, pointing out that I had to support my kids and needed this job. Well, that did the trick. I started off challenging myself. Each time I made my personal goal, I raised the bar. I ended up becoming the first person in the state to reach $100,000. When I accomplished this, I went for the region. I got it! During this time, I was asked to put together training manual on sales and deliver it to other representatives. If you know anyone who works for Verizon sales and have heard the expression, *"If they're breathing—bridge,"* that's me! I won several trips and was a multiple times member of the prestigious sales Winner's Circle and Master's Club.

From sales rep, I was promoted to trainer and six months later, to assistant manager. In 1998 I was promoted to office manager, overseeing two offices. I also decided to finish college; since I already had my associate degree in liberal arts and I had to put my education on hold to support my kids. In 2001, I finally received my BA degree from Thomas Edison State College in New Jersey. So I was on a roll. I felt the world was mine to have. I had a good family, a good high-paying job, and a good life.

During my first year with cancer, I was on disability struggling through the multiple setbacks and surgeries. After radiation, against my husband's wishes, I returned to work. Our vice president called me and asked if I could develop a sales training package to teach service representatives how to sell long distance. At this time Verizon was entering this new territory. So I, along with Nelson, whom I call a computer genius, developed a training package. We designed a T-shirt with a map that looked like a puzzle with all of the sales features on it and the slogan, "Give them all the pieces, Long Distance completes the puzzle." Later, I was given a small staff to help produce the training package. It proved to be successful. I absolutely loved this position. I was so proud of this accomplishment.

Unfortunately, the fatigue was overwhelming and my blood count dropped, so I had to leave a place I had devoted a big portion of my life to. Cancer robs you not only physically but mentally as well. It was hard for me to accept that I didn't have the same energy level that I had before. Mike said that before cancer I had an abnormally high energy level, so now I was on par with the rest of the world. He said, "You may not walk as fast as you used to, but you can still walk!" It's nice to have someone with the voice of reason.

CHAPTER FIVE

FRIENDS AND PARTNERS

I can't stress enough the importance of having friends and loved ones surrounding you. But now let's talk about the kind of friends we want. As I told you, I woke up in the hospital and found my good friend Pat smiling over me. Because she had experienced the whole regimen regarding breast cancer— mastectomy, chemotherapy, radiation, drugs—she walked me through everything. This was wonderful, because I knew what to expect. If something happened, I was able to determine whether it was normal or abnormal. She was my guardian angel throughout this, constantly calling and checking up on me. Then there were Joyce and Bev, who kept me laughing. Joyce was my "kick in the butt" whenever I felt down. She has stuck by me through the good and bad times. There wasn't a day that went by that she didn't call. My lifelong friend Renee, who is like a sister, mothered me through this whole time. She provided me with the soothing voice I needed, not to mention gave me updates on our favorite soap operas. She kept everything on a human level. Felicia called me at least three times a week and gave me the latest updates on the job. I received hundreds of flowers and cards. If you walked into my house during that time, you would have thought that I had died, with all of the flowers and plants. I was especially touched by the monthly inspirational cards I received from the vice president of Verizon.

But then I had another friend, whose name I won't mention, who cried every time she called me. Don't get me wrong—she loved me and like everyone else was scared and concerned. But the last thing I needed was someone constantly reminding me of the stage of cancer I was in and the severity of it. Every time she called, she would cry about the good times "we used to have"! I had to constantly remind her, "Hey, I'm not dead yet and don't plan on dying!" It got so bad that every time the phone rang, I checked the caller ID and refused her calls. I had to do this because no matter how much I stressed the importance of staying positive, she just didn't get it. On top of all this, when I was first diagnosed, the only person I called was my director. I had to have time to absorb the information. But you know how jobs are; it didn't take long for the word to get around. Well, she was a little upset because I didn't call her first to tell her the news. I guess she wanted to be the first one to blab.

Get rid of any negativity. It's times like this when you see who your friends and partners are. If you feel depressed or indecisive when you are around them, *get rid of them!* Attitude is everything when you are going up against cancer.

Now, I was fortunate to have a husband who encouraged me and stuck by me. But I had another friend who was facing breast cancer. Her best chance for survival was a mastectomy. Her husband didn't want her to lose her breast, so she had to "think about it"! Are you kidding me? I told her that if he really chose her breast over her life, then maybe she should choose life over him and kick him to the curb. People, men or women, when it comes to saving your life, share your decision with your partner, but don't let him or her make the decision for you.

One of my other friends had just been diagnosed with colon cancer, when she found out that her husband of twenty years was cheating on her. She called me, hysterical. She was praying that the cancer would kill her, because her husband, whom she loved and trusted, just had. When she dismissed that thought, she said she just wanted a divorce. I told her that now wasn't the time. No, I wasn't crazy. I was thinking of her. I knew the treatment she was going to have to endure and that she was going to need every bit of her strength. I knew firsthand that divorce can be very stressful. After what seemed to be endless conversations, she finally agreed. As it turned out, the cancer changed something in her husband. For the first time, he realized how important she was to him. Through counseling, they ended up saving their marriage.

Farther down the road, I am going to tell you true stories about cancer survivors and what they endured that will amaze you.

CHAPTER SIX

LOOK GOOD, FEEL EVEN BETTER

Right after my mastectomy, a nurse visited me who told me about the programs that were available to breast cancer patients at the American Cancer Society. One of them was called "Look Good, Feel Better." This was a free workshop provided by the American Cancer Society that showed you different beauty tips as to how to be beautiful after cancer. Now, I can tell you, people, after going through the mental anxiety I had to deal with—hearing that I had breast cancer, losing both breasts—the last thing I cared about was my looks. As a matter of fact, I felt like looks were a thing of the past. But as I looked in the mirror one day, examining the after effects of chemo—like losing my hair, losing my eyebrows, pale skin—I said to myself, "Yeah, you need help." So off to "Look Good, Feel Better" I went.

I was apprehensive at first when I walked into the beauty seminar. But after being there about twenty minutes, sharing war stories with other women, I started relaxing. They showed us how to apply eyeliner so that it didn't look like it was drawn on your face. In addition, we received wig tips and foundation tips, to cover that sallow look. All in all, it was a fun day. I learned a lot. I walked out of there with a gift bag of cosmetics and, shall we say, not feeling so cancerous!

I want to address the ladies out there. Girls, this isn't a vanity thing; this has a lot to do with your own personal recovery. If you look bad, you feel bad. I'm going to add, even if you don't have cancer, there is no reason on earth to let yourself go to pot as you get older. Yes, our partners are supposed to love us no matter what; but come on, ask yourself, if you looked unattractive when you met him, would he have married you? I'm not talking about full-blown plastic surgery. You would be surprised by what a little lip gloss, mascara, and blush can do. You want him to want you, not just tolerate you. Fellas, this goes for you too. Not too many women find an out-of-shape man sexy.

Now, with regard to wigs, let me give you a few tips. I have found that most of the wig and prosthetic places that advertise they cater to breast cancer patients, charge ridiculous prices—mainly because they know the insurance companies provide some reimbursement. But let me tell you a story. I went with my girlfriend to one of these places to get a wig. The prices started at $250.00. The one she picked out was a cheap-looking synthetic wig that looked like a birds' nest on her head. I've had human hair and synthetic wigs, and prices have ranged from $30.00 to $100.00. Check around. The Internet provides a lot of resources. You can always take it to a beautician to have it styled to fit your face.

Next, join an exercise class. If that's not possible, make it a point to walk every day and to do some stretching exercises. This is good for your health as well as your looks. Remember, before you hit 200 pounds, you had to pass 125 pounds. So don't let it get out of hand. Decide what weight is healthy for you, and aim for it. Now, don't get me wrong; I still treat myself to the good stuff—fried chicken, ice cream, cake, etc.—I just keep an eye on my weight.

It's also important to wear proper-fitting clothing. I know that ages have crossed paths when it comes to clothes, but make sure they fit properly. If you want to hide the lumps and bumps, go a little larger and looser. Have you ever seen a person with their clothes so tight you can count the moles on their body? Yuk!

CHAPTER SEVEN

LIFE AFTER CANCER

As I stated before, when I went back to work, I was extremely tired. My blood count never bounced back. I was still getting Procrit and Zometa treatments, but the symptoms remained. It was at this time that Mike asked me if he could get a transfer to upstate New York, whether I would move. You see, we had vacationed there often and always said that would be the place we would go when we retired. I said yes, thinking he would never get it. But low and behold, after one month of sending out his resumes, his transfer came through. It happened so fast that he had to leave before me, while I stayed and put our house on the market. On Valentine's Day 2003, I made the move.

The first couple of years, I went through withdrawal—no job, nothing to do. I was going crazy. I decided to call the American

Cancer Society and ask if they could use me in a volunteer position. That is when I met Tracy. After my interview, she suggested I become a Reach to Recovery counselor. Since I majored in psychology, it wasn't a stretch. I went through the training. I was so nervous when I took my first call. But I can't explain the overwhelming sense of accomplishment when you begin a conversation with a devastated individual, and end with laughter. In training we were always told to limit our hours of calling so that our lives were not completely overwhelmed. But I made myself available at all hours. I remember waking up in the middle of the night and wanting someone to talk to—to tell him or her how I was feeling. Many a day and night, I talked with men and women, helping them deal with their journey with cancer. Once, I took a call at midnight and stayed on the phone until 2:00 AM. You see, this person had just lost her favorite uncle, and she herself was going through treatment. So I knew how important it was to get her in the right frame of mind.

Then Tracy asked me to be the keynote survivor speaker at one of their Reach for Recovery kickoff breakfasts. I foolishly thought I would be speaking to about fifty people, but it turned out to be six hundred people. I spent days writing and rewriting my speech. Every time I practiced it in front of Mike, I would flub a line here or there. When the time came, I threw the written speech to the side and just got up there and told my story. You know what? It flowed. From there, I was asked to be in photo shoots, pertaining to cancer, for New York State and Price Chopper. I have made several guest appearances on Benita Zahn's *Health Link*, and her NewsChannel 13 Live at 5 and 6, and on radio stations. I still perform speaking engagements at the local clubs, covering all types of cancer. I can honestly say I owe Tracy so much. She brought the old Inez back to life.

But that still wasn't enough for me. When I was diagnosed with advanced cancer in 2001, I felt there weren't enough people around, in my stage of cancer, to talk to. I used to wonder if they were still with us. When I moved to upstate New York, I pondered writing a newspaper column, relaying information and stories about people—men, women, children, even animals—who have survived all stages and types of cancer. I wasted more time telling myself that I couldn't do it, rather than telling myself I could.

Then one day my life changed. I was attending a health-care day with a friend of mine, when I was fortunate to meet another cancer survivor named Bootie Fenoff. Bootie herself has an amazing story I will tell you about later. Anyway, we started chitchatting. I told Bootie about my desire to write a column, but I was fairly new to Upstate, didn't know a lot of people, and had zero experience when it came to writing a column. We discussed it awhile, with her giving me suggestions; then she left. About an hour later, Bootie returned with a gentleman in tow. She introduced him to me, told me he was a cancer survivor, and said, "He wants to give you a story; now write!" I sat there about a minute with my mouth wide open. I finally gathered my courage and started writing his story. Soon, Bootie brought a woman over who was another cancer survivor, and *bam*, another story.

I met with Ray Pignone, the managing editor of *The Catskill Daily Mail*, Catskill, New York, and pitched my idea about writing a column to encourage cancer survivors. He thought it was a good idea, but he had to discuss it with someone else. Within two weeks, "Cancer Kickin' Warriors" was born. My friend who was a computer whiz and I wrote stories about people surviving cancer and informational columns. Shortly after, she left, and I continued with the column, which is still going strong to this day. Then I was honored when Teresa Hyland, the executive editor, contacted me and asked if I wanted to run my column in *The Catskill Daily Mail*'s sister paper, *The Hudson Register-Star*, Hudson, New York. Of course I jumped at the idea. I commend *The Hudson Register-Star* and *The Catskill Daily Mail* for giving cancer survivors a voice.

My column appeared every Saturday, until I had two rotator cuff surgeries on the same side, so now it appears every other week. This column brought a lot of attention to cancer. It made people open up and talk about their ordeal with cancer. This also opened the door for more speaking engagements and more counseling. One of my friends asked me why I do all of these things when I don't get paid. My answer is simple: "God paid me in advance, and I'm alive. Now I owe him!"

When the U.S Preventive Services Task Force came up with that ridiculous recommendation about women not getting a mammogram until age fifty, I, along with Betty Betts, Bootie Fenoff, and Elba Potestas, sprang into action. We called ourselves, above all things, "The Cancer Kickin' Warriors," and we started a petition challenging this decision. Since then, we have taken up numerous cancer-related causes. We keep watch on any health-care changes. We have met with numerous politicians—People, we are serious! Betty and I have spent countless hours on our laptops poring through the new health-care bill. Let me say it's a privilege to work with these women. Betty Betts, herself a DCIS cancer survivor, Bootie Fenoff, a multiple cancer survivor, and Elba Potestas (president of the Greene County Women's League Cancer Patient Aid) are tireless, compassionate women working to help cancer patients.

I joined the Greene County Women's League Cancer Patient Aid, which is a bare-knuckle nonprofit group that provides some financial relief to people going through cancer. I now serve on their board. One day at a luncheon that Bootie attended as a guest, the ladies at the table wanted to know why I never wrote a book. I said, "Mike, my husband, has been pushing me, but I don't know how to do it."

Well, as soon as the words came out of my mouth, I heard a voice say, "You *will* write a book!" You guessed it—Bootie! And here I am, folks. Bootie, along with my husband and children, has been my anchor. Not knowing anything about writing, they have helped with a lot of research and contacts. To them I am eternally grateful.

You've heard my story; now I want to present Cancer Kickin' Warriors stories that have appeared in my column over the years.

THE WARRIORS

BOOTIE FENOFF

Have you ever felt that God put a person in your life that has a special purpose? This is the story of the most remarkable, unselfish, giving person that I know. Bootie has personally inspired me and pushed me to limits I never knew I could reach. Her own personal story will inspire you and give you the courage to conquer not only cancer, but any obstacle that may enter your life.

In March 1992, Bootie went for her routine mammogram and as always everything was fine except for some calcium deposits. In May, however, while performing her monthly self-exam, she noticed a lump on her right breast. It didn't alarm her, because she had just had a mammogram, which turned out to be clear. But this "thing" kept getting bigger. So she called her primary physician. He ordered an ultrasound, and the results came back clear. He then ordered a second mammogram; again the results came back clear. But Bootie knew her body. She insisted something was not right, so he referred her to a surgeon.

What I love about Bootie is that she is a take-charge lady. Upon seeing the surgeon, she insisted on having a biopsy. Bootie knew that something was not right. Your breast doesn't produce a continuing growing lump for no reason at all.

The surgeon performed a surgical biopsy, put a drain in, and told her to return in a week to have it removed. Just when Bootie and her husband, Dick, were literally getting ready to revisit the surgeon, her primary doctor called, asking her if she knew the results of her biopsy. Bracing herself, she heard the words we all dread to hear— it's cancer! Bootie said she felt like the room was closing in on her. But there was Dick, her rock, who told her they were not going to worry about it because she was going to conquer this. He also made it known that Bootie had to have the best doctors.

The surgeon ordered numerous tests—bone scan, heart, x-rays, etc. The tests also focused on a spot that developed on Bootie's ankle, but fortunately that came back noncancerous.

Now, folks, it's important to point out that at this time Bootie's daughter, Lori, was pregnant with Bootie's first grandchild. Bootie also has a son, Ron. She didn't know how she was going to tell them that she had cancer. Remember, this was 1992 and the word *cancer* equaled death in the minds of people. But Dick took charge and assured her he would tell the kids. Again in a calming voice, he assured them Bootie was going to get through this.

Bootie went to an oncologist, Dr. Harvey Zimbler. He discussed with her the option of having a mastectomy or lumpectomy. As always, she discussed her options with Dick. He made it clear to her that it was her decision. He told her he did not marry her for her breasts. That was not who she was. But because the surgeon felt that they could get it all with a lumpectomy, Bootie opted for that procedure.

Bootie was scheduled for the operation on July 8, 1992. Dick did not want Lori to come to the hospital, because it was close to her due date. Well, as usual, Dick was right on the money, because Lori went into labor on that very date. Her son, Tyler, was born on July 9, and for all you astrology folks out there, you know that makes his sign, of all things—Cancer! Bootie had mixed emotions. She was happy that she successfully made it through surgery, but said she was sad she had missed the birth of her first grandchild. But those mixed emotions turned to joy when her son and daughter-in-law came to the hospital with a video of her new grandson. Bootie said the nursing staff was wonderful. They scoured around till they found a VCR. People, I'm sure right now you are getting the picture of the type of marriage the Fenoffs had and the kind of man Dick was.

Now, even though the surgeon assured Bootie and Dick that he had gotten clean tissue, Dr. Zimbler scheduled a regimen of six months of chemotherapy and seven weeks of radiation. Bootie underwent both of them at the same time!

In addition, she was starting her own alteration business and taking care of her new grandson. I looked at this superwoman in sheer amazement. I had chemotherapy and radiation, and I can assure you I didn't have the will or energy to do anything. But Bootie said all of this gave her a reason to get up in the morning. She was not going to let cancer take control of her life or change the type of person she was. In six months she was declared cancer free.

So the next fourteen years passed pretty uneventfully. But in 2006, Bootie noticed a spot on the same breast where she had the lumpectomy. She went to a dermatologist, who didn't quite know what it was, so he took a biopsy. Growing alongside the original spot was another black spot the doctor was concerned about. So he took another biopsy of that the same day. Well, wouldn't you know it; it came back squamous cell carcinoma. (According to the American Cancer Society, squamous cell carcinoma is a skin cancer that develops in the upper part of the epidermis. It is more likely to spread to fatty tissues and lymph nodes.) Bootie and Dick, without a second thought, wanted the mole removed. Once the stitches were removed, the doctor wanted to be certain he had gotten it all and that the spot was clear. He did Mohs surgery.

But now, remember the original spot we talked about, which she had gone to see the dermatologist about originally— well, that test finally came back and that test was inconclusive. After several biopsies, a doctor in Albany suspected Bootie had developed T-cell lymphoma (a cancer that attacks the immune system). This type of cancer is known to attack from the waist down, but this attacked Bootie's whole body. So she began the standard treatment called PUMA. Unfortunately, Bootie suffered horrific side effects from this treatment. She had uncontrollable itching and said she burned so bad, she looked like a lobster. This was one time Bootie felt like she wanted to die! After one month of sheer torture, treatment was stopped. She went back to her doctor, who in turn referred her to the Dana-Farber Cancer Institute in Massachusetts. Here, they definitively confirmed that Bootie in fact had T-cell lymphoma. She had to undergo three more surgical biopsies in order to set up a treatment tailored to her.

After one month, a treatment was finally discovered in December. She was given Ontak, a chemotherapy drug, intravenously. It was stretched out in intervals of every three weeks, then three months, and then six months, with the prospect of her being cured in a year. But of course this is Bootie we're talking about, where things don't always go as planned. In July, Dr. Zimbler attempted to increase the interval between Ontak dosages; but she developed very prominent skin changes marked by diffuse itching. His impression was Bootie's disease was relapsing. So she was put on high doses of prednisone.

In July 2007, a beautiful love story repeated itself. Dick and Bootie Fenoff celebrated their fiftieth wedding anniversary by renewing their vows. This was peaked by a beautiful reception given by their children and grandchildren. Friends, I can tell you, their story is one that you read about. When you saw one, you saw the other. After fifty years together, they looked like two teenagers who were falling in love for the first time.

Then in September 2007, fate took an ugly, unspeakable turn. Bootie lost the love of her life. This man who had supported her, been her rock, carried her back and forth to every doctor's appointment and treatment, was now gone. This was more devastating to her than hearing she had cancer. What was she going to do without Dick? How would she get to her chemo treatments? She had supportive children, family, and friends; but Dick was the other half of her.

In 1993, Bootie along with three friends had started a cancer support group just to discuss issues concerning cancer. At one time this group had grown to as many as twenty-five members. To this day, it meets the third Tuesday of the month. When she lost Dick, her friends, family, and support group members got together and came up with a schedule to take Bootie to her treatments in Massachusetts. This gives you an idea how loved and respected this woman is. She had been there for them; now they were going to be there for her.

In January 2007 three chemo treatments were set up. In addition to Ontak, she had to orally take another chemo drug called Targretin. She took three pills daily at night.

In March 2009, Bootie noticed a black spot on her scalp.

She went to her oncologist, who referred her to a dermatologist. It was squamous cell carcinoma. Bootie's reaction was, "No, not again!" Remember she had lost her "rock"; now it was up to her alone to tell her kids she had cancer again. For those of you that are keeping track, we are now up to four bouts with cancer! Her children picked up the mantle for dad. Lori took her for another biopsy, and her son, Ron, took her for surgery. She had to see her dermatologist every six months. You would think by this time, this woman had had more than her share of tragedies. Think again.

In October 2009, while she was visiting her dermatologist, it was discovered she now had basal skin cancer; again more surgery! She also had to continue with chemotherapy, and finally on December 9, 2009, she was declared in remission.

Now you understand why I have nothing but the utmost admiration and respect for this woman. She has survived her bouts with cancer and above all, the loss of her beloved husband, Dick. If I even entertain the thought of feeling sorry for myself, I think of Bootie. After all of what she's been through, you would think she would crawl in a hole and pull the hole in after her—*Think again!*

Bootie still runs the Ghent Support Group, participates in the Columbia Healthcare Consortium's annual "Walking with Our Neighbors for Our Neighbors," is a member of our Cancer Kickin' Warriors group, and still finds time to talk to patients or family members dealing with cancer.

I asked Bootie for some words of wisdom for our fellow warriors. She says:

Regardless of what life throws at you, you can always find a happy ending.

There is a reason why we are here; find that reason.

Don't let cancer change who you are. It may set you back, but not knock you out.

Love and support are what get you through the hard times.

Believe in God; in the end he doesn't let you down.

Don't be afraid to talk about cancer. You may be saving someone else's life.

Fight. Cancer is an aggressive opponent, so you have to be just as aggressive.

If Dick Fenoff were here with us today, I would thank him for the many years of love and support he gave Bootie, for taking her to the multiple doctor's visits and treatments, for not letting her give up when she wanted to. But most of all, if Dick were here, I would thank him for the beautiful angel he left here to help other cancer warriors.

Edward C.

Men act fast, save your life

To all of our men out there, pay attention! This story may save your life.

In September 1999, fifty-eight-year-old Edward C. experienced a burning sensation when he urinated. At first he didn't pay too much attention to it, but the pain became more intense. After three days, Ed made an appointment with his doctor. At first, she suspected he had a bladder infection and began treating him with antibiotics. She told him if it was a simple bladder infection, he should see some improvement within five days.

Well, folks, that wasn't the case, so she referred Ed to an urologist, Dr. Daniel Melamed. While in the office, Ed had a scope inserted which detected tumors. From there arrangements were made to have a biopsy done. They took portions next to the wall of the bladder. Though sedated, Ed told me he watched the whole procedure! The results came back that Ed had bladder cancer. Now on top of this devastating news, Ed was told that the cancer possibly went through the wall of the bladder into other vital organs. His only path to survival was to have his bladder removed.

Ed was referred to Westchester Medical Center, which specialized in this type of surgery. His pathology report was sent ahead to the facility for examination. Now at the time, there were five options for bladder and reconstructive surgery. Ed had opted for the old-fashioned kind, where the bladder is removed and you wear a bag on the outside.

A guardian angel must have been sitting on Ed's shoulder, for about three days before the surgery he received a call stating that the cancer had not spread through the wall, so his bladder could stay intact. Ironically, Dr. Melamed's father, who was a pathologist, was the one who made this discovery! Ed said upon hearing the news, he cried. I have to tell you people, just writing this story brought tears to my eyes.

So by October back to Hudson Ed and his wife went, to have the tumor removed. It took four operations, each time removing about one-fourth of the tumor. The surgeries were scheduled about a week apart. After the second surgery, Ed had to wear a catheter, because they enlarged the urinary tube.

After surgery, Ed was put on an intravenous cocktail of CBG and interferon. Ironically, CBG is the same bacteria used in vaccinations against tuberculosis! It's administered directly into the bladder through a thin, flexible tube. Ed went once a month for months, then every three months from 2000 to 2003. During 2003–2007, his treatments were reduced to every six months. In addition, he had a scope performed every six months. I know you men may flinch at the thought of this test, but let me tell you, Ed said he sat through the whole procedure, chitchatting with the doctor.

Eureka! In April, Ed was given a clean bill of health! He now has a special urine test done once a year that detects cancer.

Ed credits his primary doctor for acting fast. She started off treating him for a bladder infection, but did not wait when antibiotics were ineffective. He praises Dr. Melamed for saving his life and the doctor's father for interpreting his report correctly, which saved his bladder.

Ed has some words for all of our men folk out there:

Don't wait; if something is not right, see your doctor, and above all act on it until the symptoms go away.

Don't be afraid, whatever the diagnosis or treatment. He said he would go through every bit of this again if it means saving his life.

Cancer does not pick and choose any one individual; no one is 100 percent safe. The main thing is if you have the slightest discomfort—check it out!

Family is everything. He said it was the love and strength of his wife, Beverly, and children that got him through a very difficult time in his life.

Folks, I wish you had the pleasure I had in talking to Edward. He is the most easygoing, soft-spoken, courageous, and delightful man. He said when he first heard he had cancer, he wasn't really nervous, because he didn't know a lot about it. He just had a will to live and was going to do whatever it took.

Fellas, I know you don't like to talk about your illnesses, but Ed's candidness about his cancer might have saved your life. He had to be brave to go through it and even braver to share his story. Edward, thank you for giving our men folk a wake-up call.

ALBERT T.

Breast cancer doesn't discriminate.

In my November article, I promised to bring the story about someone very close to me who was diagnosed with breast cancer. What makes this story so different from the many stories I write on breast cancer, is that this very special person is a man!

Recently, I had a visit from my former brother-in-law, Albert T, who has always been like a brother to me. We began chitchatting, catching up on old times, when he shocked me with the words, "Well, sis, I never told you, but I was diagnosed with breast cancer five years ago." I couldn't believe it, since Albert never even had a cold, ate healthy, and was always the picture of health. When I told him about our column, he wanted to tell the story to help other men and let them know it is not just a "woman's disease."

Albert said he had never gone to the doctors. He relied on having a healthy lifestyle—eat right, no alcohol or smoking.

This carried him for fifty years. But he decided at age fifty to have a complete physical, including a colonoscopy. The tests came out fine. He continued with the yearly checkups. But on one visit he mentioned to the doctor that he noticed a small lump around the nipple, which started to grow and itch. The doctor asked how long he had noticed it. Albert said about fifteen years!

His doctor didn't panic but suggested he see an oncologist just to rule out cancer. Albert had a biopsy, and about a week later the doctor told him he had breast cancer. I asked Albert how he felt upon hearing those words. His answer will amaze you. He said, "You know, I never flinched; I believed that God would bring me through anything. The doctor suggested surgery, and I said, 'Let's do it.'"

Three days later Albert had a mastectomy but no chemotherapy or radiation. He has almost completed his Arimidex regimen. The doctor said he had a guardian angel because that cancer stayed in one spot for all of those years, coupled with the fact that his seeing a doctor when it started to grow might have saved his life.

Albert has these words for our men folk out there:

- Breast cancer is not just a woman's disease.
- He was lucky. But examine your breast; if you feel something out of the ordinary, *see a doctor.*

- Have faith in God—cancer is not the end of the world.
- Make sure you have routine prostate and colonoscopy exams.

Oh, by the way, did I mention Albert is now seventy years old and looking good. Cancer did not slow this man down. He enjoys trips to Atlantic City and the Millennium in Pennsylvania. His family, friends, and church, and above all, God, have been a great source of strength for him. He has been working as a private-duty caregiver.

My main reason for telling Albert's story is to tell our men—know your body. Don't you be the one to raise those death statistics due to male breast cancer. Remember, my motto is, "Don't be afraid if you have cancer; be afraid if you don't do anything about it!"

BETTY B.

Did not waste time

Now we are going to travel on a journey with a dear friend of mine who fought and won her battle with DCIS. I think you may know this neighbor. I'll give you a hint; she is *the* lady of all ladies!

From the time she was forty, Betty was faithful about getting her routine mammograms. You see, not only was there a family history of cancer, but Betty also had atypical precancerous cells. Through the mammograms, two lumps were discovered in 2002 and 2005. Thankfully, they were benign. But for the next two years she diligently went every six months to have her follow-up mammogram. But then her insurance wouldn't pay, so she went one year without one.

Then in November 2007, Betty went for her yearly physical, including the mammogram. The doctor saw something suspicious, so an ultrasound and biopsy were performed. Betty received that call we all dread. She was told she had DCIS (ductal in situ carcinoma at stage I). DCIS is when the cancer is confined to the ductal glands. Betty's doctor cautioned her that the treatment usually consisted of a lumpectomy, radiation, and the removal of some lymph nodes. I asked Betty about her feelings when she heard this. She told me she was petrified. While driving, she pulled over to the side of the road and just cried.

Betty was referred to Dr. Henna, a surgeon. Betty's records were sent to him in advance. I accompanied Betty, along with her then fiancé, John, to Dr. Henna's office. He wanted to know exactly what she was told. Betty answered that she was told she had DCIS stage I. Dr. Henna then said, "No, you have stage 0; it was caught early and had not spread outside of the duct." Henna scheduled another biopsy, MRI, and finally a lumpectomy.

About one week after the lumpectomy, Dr. Henna informed Betty that it was a small tumor and the outside margins were clear. He told her she would probably not need radiation but would be put on a regimen of tamoxifen. This, however, would be up to the oncologist. Betty said she again had tears, but this time they were tears of joy. It was over! This whole ordeal took about a month.

Henna was right on the money. The oncologist referred Betty to a radiologist, who concurred that she did not need radiation. The oncologist did, however, put her on tamoxifen, and Betty continues with her mammograms. Betty points out that even though she has some joint pains due to the tamoxifen, the benefits far outweigh the side effects.

Today Betty continues to work. She is the recording secretary for the Fortnightly Club. She also performs volunteer work and is a founding member of the Cancer Kickin' Warriors Club. She divides her time between her now hubby, John, and cute-as-a-button grandson, Cayden. She is very vocal about her situation because she wants women of all ages to know that if she had not had the mammograms, which caught her cancer early, she might be telling a different story. Betty's advice is to be proactive before it advances. She said she would go through every test and procedure again, if it means saving her life. Her actions saved her breast and her life.

Betty says she couldn't have made it without her strong support team.

Her daughters, Lisa and Ashley, made themselves available whenever she needed them. Their time became Betty's time. No mother could have asked for more love, than the love she received from her beloved daughters.

Betty's then fiancé, John, was a constant fixture by her side. She says, "While Dr. Henna was explaining everything to us, I saw love, not fear, in his eyes. He is one of the most selfless, caring men that I know."

And finally, Betty praises Dr. Henna, not just because he is an outstanding surgeon, but also because he and his wife (who works with him) are very sensitive to their patients' feelings. He patiently answers all of your questions in such a calming, reassuring voice. They can not do enough for their patients.

Betty, you are my friend, my champion, and *a lady*!!

JOYCE D

Life goes on.

In the beginning of my story, I told you about my stubborn, hardheaded Sagittarian friend, who has been my rock. Joyce D. is like the sister I never had. She has always been there for me, and vice versa. So you can imagine the shock I felt when she called me and told me she was diagnosed with multiple myeloma, a cancer of the bone marrow.

In April 2008, Joyce went to her primary physician for her regular check up. When the results of her routine blood work came back, it showed her protein levels were high. Her doctor referred her to a hematologist.

The hematologist did another blood test; when those results came back, a third one was ordered. It was then she informed Joyce that she wanted to do a bone marrow test. Joyce said she wasn't concerned at this point, because she thought it was routine. Her sister accompanied her because she thought she might be a little woozy.

After three days, the doctor called with the results—Joyce had multiple myeloma. The hematologist explained this was a slow-moving cancer. Thankfully, she probably would not need any advance treatment for about ten years. The first year of diagnosis, Joyce had a blood test every four months. The second year it was reduced to every three months, and now it's back to a blood test every four months. Joyce says the reason for the change in year two, is because she takes prednisone to manage it and the doctor wanted to see if this caused any change. Fortunately, she says the disease has not had any serious impact one her.

I asked her about her feelings when she was told she had cancer. She said in regard to herself, she had no immediate feeling. She accepted it, did her research, and put her faith in God's hands. She said she was more concerned about her family and friends. At first she didn't want to tell them, because she didn't want them to worry. Folks, I know this lady, and believe me she's telling the truth. She always puts other people first. We worked together, and she was always the take-charge, go-to person, putting everyone else first. Aside from being smart, she has a wit about her that will keep you laughing anytime you're with her.

She has some words of wisdom for other cancer warriors:

+ Just because you have cancer, your world doesn't have to end.

- Cancer is not a death sentence. As she puts it, "I can leave my house tomorrow and get killed in a car accident."
- Live your life. Don't let cancer consume you.

People, no multiple myeloma or any cancer is going to get this warrior down!

ARLENE O.

A new treatment

In February 2009, Arlene went for her yearly mammogram. Her doctor was concerned about the images, so a second one was ordered along with an ultrasound. These results still looked suspicious, so Arlene's doctor performed a needle biopsy.

After three days Arlene received a call, at night no less, from her doctor. Now we know a doctor calling at night with test results is usually pretty serious, and it was. The tests detected breast cancer. At the time Arlene said after hearing those words, she didn't hear anything else. Fortunately, James, her husband of forty-nine years (that's a story in itself, guys), was sitting beside her reading the expression on her face and watching her eyes welling up with tears. When she told him about the results of the test, he was the calming voice of reason. James assured her he would be by her side and together they would get through this. Arlene also has two sons. One was in the navy and at sea during this time. She opted not to tell him anything at that moment, because there was nothing he could do except worry. Now, folks, it's important to note that neither the doctor nor Arlene could feel the lump. If it wasn't for the mammogram, a bad situation could have been worse.

Then Arlene, along with her daughter-in-law, who is a nurse, went to the doctor. The decision was made to have a lumpectomy. They also removed lymph nodes, which fortunately were clean. It was discovered she was in an early stage of cancer—stage I. This was now March, so you can see no time was wasted. Now, people, here is where we learn something new. Arlene had two follow-up choices. She could have chemotherapy along with conventional radiation. This would involve receiving radiation every day for seven weeks. The side effects usually include sunburn-like skin and fatigue. The other option, which was the one she chose, was to undergo a fairly new procedure, which has been around since 2002, called mammosite radiation.

In this procedure, Arlene had a balloon with a portacath surgically implanted. For one week she would go twice a day, in the AM and PM, and have the radiation directly administered through the port. Prior to each dosage, she had to have a CAT scan to make sure the device was still in place. Afterward, the balloon and the port were removed. The skin was cosmetically intact, and she experienced no side effects, and best of all, no chemo. Arlene sees her doctor, Dr. Savage, every six months to check the site. She has her blood checked by Dr. De Marco every six months. Arlene also orally takes the anti-cancer drug Arimidex daily.

Arlene wanted to especially praise the wonderful doctors and nurses who treated her. She says Dr. Duncan Savage is warm, compassionate, takes time with her, and answers all of her questions. The same is true for Dr. De Marco, who is very thorough and makes sure her patient has a full understanding of anything discussed. Arlene said she never feels "rushed through a visit." She also commends the staff of St. Peter's Hospital, where she received the mammosite treatment. In Arlene's own words, "They couldn't do enough to make me feel comfortable."

Then there is her family and above all—James. He never let fear overcome her. She believed him when he stood "rock solid" by her and said everything was going to be all right. Hey, folks, I told you they've been married forty-nine years; need I say more?

As I always do, I asked Arlene for her words of wisdom. She says:

+ Be diligent about getting a mammogram routinely. Remember neither her nor her doctor felt a lump. It was picked up through the routine screening.
+ It's so important to have caring doctors and medical staff.

• Support of spouse, family, and friends means so much.

Arlene says she feels fine now. She considers herself lucky to have caught it in time. She is enjoying life, and having fun being a grandmother to two adorable boys.

* A little extra note: the mammosite therapy is given to women who are in the early stage of cancer, have had a lumpectomy, had no positive lymph nodes, had a tumor less than three centimeters, and are over forty-five years old.

MARISOL D.

Alternative treatment

Have you ever been hit with a devastating event in your life and you don't know how to handle it? Then it seems out of nowhere God sends you a "guardian angel". That helps you through the rough times. I want to share a story about my own "guardian angel" and inspiration—Marisol D.

I was devastated when I was diagnosed with stage 3B breast cancer in 2001. Then through a mutual friend I met Marisol at a healing mass, which she still attends weekly. Upon reading her story, I believe you too will be inspired and have the will to fight any form of this deadly disease.

In 2000, Marisol was experiencing seizures, severe headaches, and vomiting. A stereotactic biopsy was performed, and Marisol was given the results—she had brain cancer. The tumor was a glioblastoma that was inoperable. Marisol recalled her initial reaction was numbness and then anger. The doctor advised her to go home and get her affairs in order, for she was terminal and had about six months to live. She immediately snapped back to the doctor, "Well, you're terminal too; we're all going to die." Looking back, Marisol realizes her anger was more of a defense mechanism.

When Marisol returned home, her family was waiting for her. They already knew the biopsy results. Needless to say, they greeted her with tears and hugs. Marisol felt as if she was walking into her own funeral. At that point her husband, Chandler, told her to go out with her two sisters and he would "hold down the fort at home."

Marisol and her sisters went to a café, where they dealt with their pain by crying and stuffing themselves with tiramisu. Afterward, they were going to go to an army/navy store to get fatigues for Marisol, she felt if she was going to be bald, she was going to have the whole GI Jane look! But then something happened that changed her direction.

Her sister had to stop at a shop called Middle Earth, to pick up some rocks for her daughter's school project. While there, they happened to hear a customer asking for a certain type of crystals to heal his ailing wife. Marisol's older sister was intrigued. She immediately went to the shopkeeper and told her about her sister's cancer diagnosis. Thinking her sister could die, she was desperate to find a cure. This surprised Marisol because they, being devout Catholics, did not believe in this, and in fact Marisol was afraid it might be "voodoo."

The shopkeeper explained there was nothing spooky about natural cures. She called them "God's pharmacy." She introduced Marisol to a Dr. Vega who practiced holistic medicine. Much to Marisol's surprise, the doctor was also Catholic!

Even though Marisol still had her reservations, she really felt guided toward this treatment. So she told her doctor, the one who told her she only had about six months to live, she was going to forgo chemotherapy and try the alternative. Over the next eight years, Marisol went through the following regimen:

- Macrobiotic diet
- Acupuncture and reflexology
- Herbal injections and supplements
- Hyperbaric oxygen therapy (cancer does not like oxygen)
- Energy work (same concept as magnets for healing)
- Breuss protocol (to starve cancer of glucose and protein)

Marisol continues her treatment with Dr. Kokayi of the Kokayi Holistic Center in New York City. I must admit, I was skeptical at first of alternative treatments. But how do I argue with someone who was originally given six months to live and is alive today, eight years later, telling her story?

When I asked Marisol what advice she could give to people, she said:

- I am still here by the grace of God, so have faith and never give up.
- Eat right, juice daily, build your immune system.
- Be careful about what you put in your body.
- Change your lifestyle (for example, she'll use an earpiece instead of holding a cell phone to her ear).
- Get rid of any negative energy (including people).
- Comedy cures, so laugh a lot.
- In the words of our dear friend, Fran Tobin, "Death will be our finest moment, so don't be afraid to live."

Folks, I'm sure you can see how this warrior gave me inspiration and expanded my thinking. Marisol, we thank you so much.

Folks, I spoke to Marisol, saying, "Let's change those eight years into ten!" She is still going strong, still kickin' cancer!

KIM P.

Strength beyond belief

Get ready to read about an amazing woman who exemplifies the words *strength, courage, faith,* and *endurance.* After interviewing this unbelievable woman, I made a personal vow to never, ever complain about anything again.

On September 11, 2004, Kim's husband walked out on her after twenty-five years of marriage. On October 11, 2004, her only child, Jared, was killed in an automobile accident. As if this wasn't enough, Kim was diagnosed with stage 2 breast cancer on December 13, 2004, and lost her beloved mother and uncle to cancer in 2005. While I was interviewing this woman, I kept saying to myself, *this can't be real.* But folks, trust me—it's real.

Horrific events hit Kim back-to-back and from all angles. She said after the loss of her son, she didn't think or feel like she wanted to fight cancer. She felt like her world was falling apart, taking everything she loved and cared about. It took a trip to specialists in Vermont, in order to get a second opinion, to snap her into the reality that she had to fight. And remember, this warrior had to fight without the people we want most around us—our spouse, our children, and our parents.

At first, Kim was going to have a bilateral mastectomy. But after further tests and under the advice of her physicians, she decided on a lumpectomy. Eight rounds of chemotherapy and seven and a half weeks of radiation followed.

Kim wants to emphasize that during her treatment, she wanted some sense of normalcy in her life. So amazingly, she continued her exercises and weekly trips to the gym. Although she was enduring excruciating emotional pain, she kept her appearance up and willed herself to keep going. She even performed volunteer work for the cancer society.

Then in 2006, Kim's life took an unexpected turn for the better. She met a wonderful man, who brought the much-needed love and support to her life. Women often ask me how to introduce the subject of cancer when you begin dating someone. Before Kim met her new man, having a relationship was the last thing on her mind. Remember, because of the rapid series of events, she never even got the chance to grieve the loss of her son. But Kim was very candid about her experience. She said she just came right out and told him everything. When the relationship got to the point of intimacy, she was more concerned about his feelings. But he recognized how wonderful and special this woman was. The way she handled her personal challenges only enhanced his opinion of her rather than diminished it. Her story also points out the importance of having someone love you and stand by you. Anyone can love you when things are going great; but when challenges hit, there lies the true test of a relationship.

In such a short time, Kim has gone through more challenges than some of us will ever endure in a lifetime, yet she is still standing. She spends much of her time performing volunteer work for the cancer society and keeping her dynamic shape intact by working out at the gym. Though she and her boyfriend are no longer together, she has no regrets. Kim says, "For every season, there's a reason." He came at the right time in her life. She is also a Reach to Recovery volunteer counselor. In 2007, she had the honor of cutting the ribbon at the opening of the Albany American Cancer Society breast cancer walk. She has that strong "survivor personality" that even she isn't aware of. Throughout this interview there was not even a hint of self-pity. Kim wants to write about her experiences to encourage people to fight and, above all, to believe in themselves no matter what happens. The happiness she shared with her man furthered her belief that "life is worth living."

As you can imagine, Kim relived a lot of pain telling us her story. But she said it was well worth it if she could make a difference and give someone else hope and strength.

Kim, we thank you and applaud you. But above all, follow that dream and write that book. I think we're looking at a future best seller.

LILY D.

Our young warrior

It seems like our warriors are getting younger, tougher, and braver. This is the story of one heck of a young lady that fits that description.

In 2003 eleven-year-old Lily wasn't feeling well. Based on her symptoms, she was diagnosed with strep throat. But after bruises developed on her body, accompanied with pain, a series of blood tests were performed. The results were not good—Lily was diagnosed with leukemia! Leukemia is a cancer of the blood, whereby the white cells reproduce at such an aggressive rate they inhibit the growth of red cells.

As a result of this diagnosis, Lily was admitted to Albany Medical Center, where for five weeks she received chemotherapy and underwent spinal taps and bone marrow biopsies.

And it was not easy by a long shot. She developed high fevers for which she was given high doses of antibiotics. She would come home for two weeks only to return and go through the same regimen again!

Lily, at the time a sixth-grader, returned to school in September. Aside from the routine visits to her doctor, she thought the worst was behind her, so she was ready to go full steam ahead with her life. The town of Coxsackie was nothing short of amazing—holding fund benefit dinners, talent shows, and raffles in support of Lily.

But then in April 2004, Lily's world was turned upside down again. After a series of blood tests, it was revealed the leukemia had returned. Lily said her initial thoughts were *I'm going to die.* Remember, folks, this is an eleven-year-old girl we're talking about. She knew this time was going to be tougher, for she needed a bone marrow transplant. Amazingly, her mom was a match. What better gift can a parent give a child than the gift of life for the second time?

Prior to the procedure, Lily had to cleanse her system and again go through intensive chemotherapy and radiation. She remained in the hospital for six weeks. If this wasn't enough, the chemotherapy she received prior to her transplant had destroyed the lining of her stomach, whereby she couldn't eat and had to be fed through a feeding tube.

Now is the time to ask, "How is Lily doing now?" Well, you be the judge. I called Lily and was greeted with that familiar upbeat, engaging voice. She told me she goes to her doctor every six months for a checkup and she is in good health. She is in the eleventh grade now and has quite a busy life. Lily is the coach for a program called "Battle of the Books" at the library. Her team consists of students in grades six through nine. Each student is given ten books to read throughout the summer. They meet once a week to discuss the books. In the fall they will compete with other teams throughout upstate New York, whereby the teams will be asked questions about the books. Lily has been involved with this for three years and has been a coach for two. She is also the only student on the building advisory committee at Coxsackie Athens High School. They are presently looking at space for new construction. And like any other teen, she has a favorite musician—Keith Greene. Lily shared a wonderful experience she had recently. While she was attending a weekly prayer meeting, the piano player approached her and asked, "Aren't you Lily D?" At that point Lily realized this was a nurse who had cared for her while she was in the transition unit for her bone marrow transplant four years ago. Lily was surprised that the nurse remembered her. But, folks, we aren't, are we? I think we can agree Lily is an unforgettable person.

As far as the future, she has her eye on one goal—Lily wants to be an oncologist specializing in treatment and research. Lily confidently states, "I'm going to find a cure for cancer!"

Folks, this heroic sixteen-year-old can teach us all a lesson. If you have faith in God, love and support of family and friends, and a strong will, you can endure anything and accomplish anything. As a cancer survivor myself, I'm holding Lily to her promise of finding a cure for cancer. Lily, God bless you and your family.

* Just an added note: Lily is now eighteen years old. She still is doing Battle of the Books and will be attending Clarkson University. She is studying biomolecular science. Lily we will be waiting for that cure!

MARGARET W.

A professor of experience

I wish I had this lady to talk to when I was diagnosed with cancer. If there was ever a story about hope and life after cancer, it's the story of Margaret W. Ironically; she was a teacher, and believe me when I say we have a lot to learn from her.

In 1964, Margaret's appendix burst, which caused her to almost lose her life. She was even given the last rites. At this time this forty-year-old newlywed was home recuperating when she crossed her arms and leaned on the windowsill, as she watched her husband, David, go to work. It was at this time she felt a lump on her right breast.

Since she was still under the care of her surgeon, due to the appendectomy, she made an appointment to see him. Everything went fast from that point on. The surgeon ran tests and admitted Margaret into the hospital for a biopsy. Margaret remembers signing a form basically giving permission that if cancer was discovered, they would perform a mastectomy. Unfortunately, that was the case. Remember, folks, this was 1964, when the standard treatment for breast cancer was a radical mastectomy. Fortunately, when her lymph nodes were removed, they came back clear of cancer. Margaret followed with the then, fairly new, cobalt radiation treatment. There were no anti-cancer drugs, like tamoxifen, at that time.

I asked Margaret about her feeling at this time, hearing she had cancer. She said she wasn't really scared, simply because she didn't know a lot about cancer. No one in her family had it or talked about it. Margaret also said because she almost died from appendicitis, nothing seemed to scare her after that. She had a whole new outlook on life.

For the next sixteen years, Margaret continued with her annual mammograms. Calcifications were discovered on her left breast, so they kept an eye on it. One of the mammograms revealed an abnormality, so Margaret went in for a surgical biopsy. While she was in the recovery room, the surgeon came in and said, "I have good news and I have bad news. The bad news is it is cancer, but the good news is we can remove it and you won't have to have chemo or radiation." So Margaret had another mastectomy.

I asked Margaret how she got through being hit twice with cancer. First, above all, she credits her husband, David, who was wonderful. Remember, folks, Margaret's ordeal started when they had only been married for a year. Talk about the test of love! She said although he was in complete shock, he became her rock. He was loving and supportive—David couldn't do enough for her. He is still standing with her after all of these years. Second, Margaret said she kept a positive attitude. She remembered the first time she was in the hospital; she shared a room with a woman who had back surgery. She was visited by her sisters-in-law, who had had mastectomies. Margaret remembered they were always dressed to the nines, were upbeat, and had a sense of humor. She attributes her positive attitude to them. They gave her encouragement.

Now after all of this, this beautiful lady did not let two bouts with cancer slow her down. As I stated, Margaret was a teacher. But since her retirement, this woman has worked with Meals on Wheels, served on the board of the Department of Aging, was trustee of the library, was a substitute teacher, was president of the Greene County Women's League Cancer Patient Aid, was a member of the Tannersville public health organization, and was on the board of the historical society. I can tell you firsthand that at eighty-six years old, Margaret has no intentions of slowing down.

Now, what have we learned here?

- First, women need to start getting mammograms and self breast exams at age forty.
- Second, there is life after cancer.

- Live your life; keep a positive attitude.
- Keep a sense of humor.
- Keep your looks up.
- Have a loving partner.

Margaret, you are one heck of a teacher and lady. You have taught us so much.

Mary S.

A saint walks among us.

We all know that as survivors, we have our good days and bad days. We have our ups and our downs. Sometimes the trials and tribulations we go through cause us to forget that there is a whole other world out there that we have to reacquaint ourselves with. Recently, I met a true "saint" who is well aware of this—Mary

Mary and her husband, Stan, have raised two biological children and one adopted, who are now adults. In addition, they are now raising four adopted Ukrainian siblings and another son named Kareel.

While Mary was going through the process of adopting Kareel, she and her husband went for a routine colonoscopy. They planned to go on a family outing afterward, so they took the kids with them. Much to everyone's dismay, this did not turn out to be routine. The doctor immediately came out and told Mary she had a mass on her colon. As if that wasn't enough, the doctors thought it had metastasized (spread) to her liver and right hip. Mary was immediately scheduled for a PET scan and CAT scan (imaging used to detect cancer) and blood work.

As I explained, Mary was in the process of adopting Kareel. Kareel has Treacher Collins syndrome, a cranial-facial malformation. He has no cheekbones, small earlobes, and a cleft palate. In addition to the phenomenal cost and paperwork for his adoption, Mary and Stan would also be facing multiple surgeries for Kareel's illness.

Mary was now facing a dilemma: should I go through this adoption, knowing what I am up against with colon cancer? Facing surgery, Mary consulted her doctor for his help in getting an answer to this question. His response was "If the Lord takes you to it, he'll bring you through it." In addition, much to Mary's surprise, her surgeon said, "This little boy will bring you through it." So Mary continued with the adoption.

On September 2, she went through surgery to remove part of her intestines. On a happy note, she was cleared of any cancer in her liver and hip. Mary had fifteen lymph nodes removed, which were also cancer free, and the mass was smaller than they originally thought. She followed with six months of oral chemotherapy.

She originally had to see her oncologist every three to four months, but now it is every two years.

Mary credits her survival not only to the Lord, but also to

the many family members and friends that gave her emotional and financial support. And of course there was Kareel. Her mission to save this child encouraged her to save herself. Mary believes in God and that there is a lot of good in life. Her advice to everyone is to spend time with your family and loved ones and have a "merry heart." Mary was the guest speaker at our recent Wellness Day sponsored by the Columbia Healthcare Consortium.

I think you now see why I referred to her as a "saint."

Mary and Stan unselfishly chose not to break up a family, so they adopted four siblings. Then they adopted a child with severe medical needs, all of the while Mary was dealing with her own medical crisis.

Even though we may go through many devastating trials in our lives, once we get through them, let us not forget to turn around and give a helping hand to someone else.

* I spoke to Mary recently, and she is doing fine. That heart of her and Stan's continues to grow.

STAN S.

Another saint

Last time, we told you the story about a remarkable woman named Mary S.

If you recall, Mary had battled colorectal cancer, while raising five adopted children—one suffering from a rare illness. Now we want to give you part two of this amazing family, Mary's husband, Stan .

Stan worked for twenty years as a clam digger on south Long Island. Needless to say, he was exposed to severe sun rays. Stan took all of the precautions, such as wearing protective clothing and sunscreen

Surprisingly, the one area he missed was his lip! Stan noticed a sore inside his lip that was not healing. His wife, Mary, was unaware of this, because it was not visible to the naked eye.

Stan finally consulted his physician, who in turn referred him to a dermatologist. Recognizing the familiar appearance of the lesion, the doctor sent him to a plastic surgeon who confirmed that a biopsy was needed. You guessed it—skin cancer!

Stan was given two choices: remove the lip or cut out the cancer. Stan opted for the latter. He had one-third of his lip removed and underwent reconstruction. He then followed with treatment to kill precancerous cells. Stan faithfully goes for his yearly checkups. To help with the chapped lips he may receive in the winter as a result of the cold weather, he uses liquid nitrogen on his lips.

It was Stan's quick observation and follow-up that saved his life. He tells anyone, "Don't ignore your body." Who would think such a small area as the lip could be affected? This demonstrates just how powerful the sun rays are!

Like his wife, Mary, Stan is a remarkable, caring, unselfish person. He didn't let this monster called cancer stop him from giving a life to five wonderful children. They are still going through their trials with their son Kareel, who has Treacher Collins syndrome—a deformity of the face. But they wouldn't trade their life for anything. This is such an inspirational, loving couple. He also credits God and a strong support group with his recovery.

Folks, there is a serious message here, especially for all of you sun worshippers out there. Is getting that golden tan worth risking your life, especially when there are so many safe tanning creams on the market and you can be any color that you want to be? Skin cancer, like many cancers, can be cured if caught early. But why go through the terror and sometimes agonizing treatments if you can possibly avoid it?

Young people, *you are not immune!*

This is one cancer that does not practice age discrimination.

RENEE A.

Stood up against colon cancer

We've heard from our warriors who are fighting and winning the war against breast cancer; now hear the story of how a young mother stood her ground and fought stage 3 colon cancer!

Renee's story began in the summer of 2004. She noticed that her energy was depleting—she was constantly napping all the time. In the fall of that same year, she noticed bleeding and was experiencing pain under her right rib. As we all do, self-diagnosing herself, she thought she had gallstones. A trip to her doctor and a colonoscopy later proved this not to be the case. Renee was initially diagnosed with stage 4 colon cancer. Her mom, who was with her at the time for support when she received the news, was, to say the least, devastated. Renee didn't want to alarm her mom by showing any emotion, so she took her hand and said, "Don't worry. Everything is going to be all right." Like any survivor will tell you, our first reaction is to portray strength to protect our loved ones from the terrible news. But like any other survivor, Renee was crushed inside.

Prior to even knowing she had cancer; Renee always said that if she ever were told she had cancer, she would refuse treatment and just wait to die. However, when it actually happened to her, she looked at her son, who was two at the time, and said, "Oh, no! I'm not leaving him." This mother was ready to take cancer on full force.

She began her chemotherapy regimen, but after two treatments she had to stop because it affected her heart. Still this feisty lady was not giving in to this monster called cancer. She decided to go the homeopathic route, using all-natural herbs and foods. She received what she calls a small gift when she learned she had stage 3, not stage 4, cancer. Like Renee says, "Hey, I'll take it."

Her doctors said that her type of cancer took about ten years to manifest itself. Thinking back, Rene recalls having pains and problems when she was in her twenties and wonders if these were warning signs of what was yet to come.

We're happy to say this beautiful lady is thriving and making other people beautiful; Rene is a beautician. This ordeal has taught Rene a lot about herself. She says she now takes better care of herself and enjoys and appreciates life even more.

* Update: Renee is still working and doing fine. She is happy to say she has had no major setbacks. She continues to enjoy life with her husband and son.

PEGGY C.

As told by her beloved daughter, Sarah

This is a story of the power of love and strength of one family. There are so many lessons we can learn.

In August of last year, my parents went on a vacation trip to the ocean. My father took my mother out to dinner, and afterward my mother realized her arms and ankles were itchy. She scratched for days thinking that it was an allergic reaction, and then before we could realize it, she developed jaundice. Jaundice is the yellowing of the skin, eye whites, and mouth gums. Her stomach hurt when she ate, when she didn't eat, when she moved, and when she didn't move. Just living day to day was a struggle for my mother. Mind you, my mother is not the type of person to sit when her feet hurt; she just walks everything off. My father and the whole family watched as my mother lost weight and became more and more sick. After a month of watching my mother fight herself being sick, we finally talked her into going to the nearest emergency care.

Scans and tests were done, and after a week or two the results came back: my mother had a blockage in the common bile duct, and in order for my mother to become healthy again, the blockage had to be removed to allow the bile to exit the body. More scans were done to see how the blockage was going to be removed.

According to the doctors, first, the blockage was a gallstone. Then it was a tumor but not cancerous. Finally, after we had all gotten over the fact that surgery would be the only way to remove it, the doctors took a final test that showed that the tumor was indeed cancerous. I think, even to this day, the hardest thing for my mother is telling her family how she is feeling and what the next step is for the treatment. The second hardest thing for all of us was and is trying so hard to not resent the doctors for not putting the twelve years of college to use to properly diagnose my mother. The absolute hardest thing for all of us to handle was when the doctors told my mother that with chemotherapy and treatment, she'd live a maximum of two years. Without treatment, she would live for six months. For anyone who hasn't thought about personally being given a death sentence, having someone you love be given one is worse than you could ever imagine. Instinctively we all imagined our lives without the rock my mother is.

Common bile duct cancer is a very rare form of cancer, and the Whipple procedure (surgery where part of the stomach, small intestine, common bile duct, and gall bladder are removed) is more complex than brain surgery. The tumor was directly between her liver and pancreas, which was helpful in removing the tumor. It also meant that none of the stomach, liver, or pancreas had to be removed in surgery.

While my mother was waiting for surgery, a plastic stent was inserted through her mouth via scope two different times and collapsed both times. Finally, a metal one was inserted, also via scope, and that involves having a metal detector card so that every time she went anywhere she'd have to have the card. This frightened her only because her life was changing and making things hard for her and the people around her. She didn't realize that we loved her enough to forget about a stupid little card.

When time came for surgery, as nervous as she was, my mother held her family together, along with herself. Five hours of surgery only brought the horrifying result that the doctors told my father: The tumor is too large and encased in veins, making it too hard to cut out without the risk of allowing the cancerous cells into the bloodstream. Although they took out her gall bladder, which was also a problem, they did not remove the cancer.

After her surgery, she had to undergo chemotherapy (pills) and radiation sent directly to her stomach, which rendered her absolutely horrified. She felt sick; she felt sick that she felt so sick; she felt horrible that she couldn't do anything; she felt horrible that she felt horrible that she couldn't change it. Cancer is to blame for this horrible time in life that my mother had. Cancer is to blame for how my mother felt, how she didn't feel, how she wished that she felt.

My mother underwent her second surgery. After nine hours of surgery and the worst day of my family's life, my mother was a warrior. When the doctors wheeled her through the hallways, my father jumped in her pathway and wanted to know how things went. When the nurse asked who he was, my mother looked up, smiled, and asked if the doctors got all of it; she cried and squeezed his hand.

My mother is one of the strongest people that I know. She will always be a hero. If cancer can't knock her down, then nothing in this world can.

I love my family for simply accepting cancer into our home, but not accepting cancer to take our mother away. I love all of the teachers, police officers, family friends, and even the people we don't even know who went out of their way to support my mother and to do whatever they could to help. I love my father for standing by my mother through all of this; it has only made their bond stronger. Finally, I love my mother for being a role model, a rock for our whole family, for being one of the strongest people I know. Mom, I love you very much, and I am so proud of you!

* People, so often I try to stress how important family is. I could not or have not made this point stronger than Sarah

and her family. Sarah took our hand and walked us through every emotion and pain her mother went through, but they still viewed her as the strength and the hero of the family. I look on Sarah and her family with such pride and admiration. For all of you warriors out there struggling with cancer and family issues, show them this story. Sarah, what you, Peggy, and your family went through, to me you are all—Cancer Kickin' Warriors!

TINA G.

You're never too old.

Recently, I had the pleasure of meeting a woman who was so positive, upbeat, and vivacious, she inspired me. This impressive lady is Tina G. For those of you who live in the area, the name may be very familiar to you. Tina was a substitute teacher for the Catskill High School for nineteen years, before retiring last year.

Prior to this, Tina worked for the New York City school system. Her love and devotion for children caused her to set up a program for special education children. In her program, she taught them the food preparation trade. She held class once a week, and then they were allowed to test their skills by working in the cafeteria.

Tina and her husband traveled extensively until 1995, when he passed away.

In 1998, through self-examination, Tina noticed a lump about the size of a pea on her left breast. She immediately went to the doctor, who performed a needle biopsy on her. She heard the words we all love to hate—she had breast cancer! Due to its size, approximately 1.5 centimeters, Tina had the option of getting a lumpectomy. Because she lost her beloved father to lung cancer, she said she would not rest unless she got it all out, so she opted for a mastectomy. Her primary doctor agreed with her.

She was scheduled to go in for surgery in May; but as fate would have it, her appendix ruptured, and she ended up with a different surgery—appendectomy. Her recovery period for this was May 23 to July 2.

In July, she had her mastectomy, and this feisty woman by her own choice only stayed in the hospital overnight.

Throughout this time, Tina had the love and support of her two daughters and loving friends.

What amazed me the most about this woman was her attitude about her ordeal with cancer. She, like most of us when diagnosed, thought she was going to die. She asked her doctor, "How long do I have?"

He said, "I don't know."

Her response was, "Good, then I am going back to college!" And that's just what she did. In 2001, this mother and grandmother of two got her degree in communications and media!

That year she was celebrated as one of the oldest people to get their degree.

Tina's message is, if you've got cancer, get rid of it. She said she's done for everyone else; now she's going to do for herself. Cancer was not going to stop her. She told me her one goal, which she will fulfill, is to write a book. Her message is "Be positive; life does go on after cancer."

As you can guess, her attitude has inspired many people. She lives the message that you can do whatever you want, no matter what obstacles are thrown at you. It's all in the attitude.

*Just an added note: I talked to Tina recently. She is now eighty-six years old! Her book is complete and ready to go to print. This proves, folks, you're never too old.

Candace R.

Don't forget to take care of yourself.

In the spring of 2006, Candace was hit with devastating news. Her husband, George, of thirty years was diagnosed with a major heart problem that required a replacement of the aortic valve. They spent the next month going to one doctor after the other getting test after test. To further complicate things, her husband did not want to get the surgery, but a second opinion confirmed that it was surgery or die.

In the midst of all the turmoil, Candace went to her doctor for her routine exam. She had canceled her appointment twice, so she felt she would hurry up and get it over with. But it proved not to be that simple. Her doctor discovered a lump and ordered a mammogram. The mammogram proved to be inconclusive, but her doctor wanted to do an ultrasound. Against her doctor's insistence, she wanted to put it off because, as she put it, her time and mind were devoted to her husband.

She never told her husband about her condition, because she didn't want him to worry.

In June her husband had his aortic valve replaced. The operation was a success. During this time her doctor called to remind her of the ultrasound. Again Candace put it off, since her husband had a difficult recovery. But one day he asked her how her exam turned out, and she casually mentioned the doctor's concern. Well, her husband was strong enough to "hit the roof." His exact words were, "You took care of me; now take care of yourself!"

Candace had the ultrasound, followed by a surgical biopsy. She not only had breast cancer, she had advanced to stage 3. She was told her best chance for survival was a mastectomy. Now she was the one to waver. But her husband, George, said, "If you can live with my new heart, I can live with your new breast." Looking back, Candace said she realized why she stayed married to this man for thirty years.

Candace had the surgery and reconstruction, followed with chemotherapy and radiation.

They also performed surgery on her other breast to even her out. She says she feels like a twenty-year-old. She told me that she and George cherish every day. They now do things that they put off for so long. Life is too short; you may not get that second chance! Her words of wisdom are, don't put off care of your own health. She would have been of no use to George if she had died.

MARVEL W.

Thanks God for dentures

Marvel's dentures may have saved his life. Marvel was experiencing pain in his mouth, predominately in the cheek. Against his wife's suggestion he continued to ignore it, coating his mouth with Anbesol. But then he noticed that he had problems with his dentures. The problem got so bad; he resorted to eating softer foods. Marvel had a strong affection for steak, so it was this that finally caused him to see a dentist.

Upon examination and hearing the symptoms, Marvel's dentist suspected something else was going on, so he referred him to an otolaryngologist (an ear, nose, and throat doctor). This specialist performed a series of tests, including a biopsy. The results were that Marvel had stage T1 oral cavity cancer. Even though Marvel's cancer had a 96 percent survival rate, you can imagine just hearing the word *cancer* threw him into a panic.

Marvel and his wife, Wilma, wanted the cancer "out," so they opted on surgery (tumor resection) followed by radiation. His only side affect was pain, which was acceptable to him compared to the alternative.

I asked Marvel about his feelings during this time. First, he said he had an overwhelming feeling of guilt, because for years, Wilma had begged him to stop smoking his pipe. He wrongly felt that because it wasn't cigarettes, it wasn't as harmful. Second, he was scared. He never understood the impact of hearing the word *cancer*, no matter how small the tumor, until it hit him!

It has been five years, and Marvel jokingly says his dentures saved his life. By the way, he got new ones.

KRIS M.

Rare, doesn't make it impossible to beat

We have heard many heroic stories from our warriors that have survived breast, lung, and prostate cancer. Well, I am proud to introduce you to a new warrior that has come forward to share her heroic story about a rare form of cancer.

In August 2007, Kris was seeing a hematologist for joint pain. At this time, she was also experiencing persistent tightness in the chest and severe pain. Not sure of the reason, her doctor wanted to prescribe medication; but knowing her body as well as she did, Kris insisted further testing be done to find the problem. So he arranged for a CAT scan.

Later that evening, she received a call from her doctor saying that her chest was fine; but it looked like a tumor was on her kidney. So another CAT was ordered, this time adding the pelvic and abdominal area. A few days later her doctor called stating that he wanted to refer her to an urologist. He never mentioned cancer, but did say if it was necessary to remove a kidney a lot of people survive well with one kidney.

When the urologist reviewed the scan, he conferred with his associates and all agreed that due to the location of the tumor, Kris needed it removed completely. You see, the tumor was located inside the kidney near her vital organs.

I asked Kris about her feelings during this time. She said at this point she wasn't scared, because of the wonderful support team she had, which included her husband, Chris, mother, and in-laws. The anxiety set in when she was preparing to have surgery on October 1, and the night before they called to tell her it had been postponed until October 15. Kris said it was just the thought of the cancer growing inside her while she was waiting that drained her emotions!

On October 15, she had the surgery. She awoke to eleven loving people surrounding her. She felt everything was going to be all right from this point on. But it wasn't until her first follow-up visit that the enormity of the situation finally hit her.

The doctor's said that her type of kidney cancer was very aggressive and not very responsive to chemotherapy. But there was hope. He suggested she participate in a trial that went as follows:

- Go once a week for six months for an infusion.
- She wouldn't know if she was getting the drug that detected cancer and killed it, or a placebo.

- It was a five-year study. She had a CAT scan every three months for two years.
- Then the remaining three years she would have a CAT scan every six months.

She just finished her last infusion. A scan revealed small spots. Kris went to a thoracic surgeon, who said they were too small to biopsy. Good news, however—when he did another scan three months later, the spots were gone.

Kris is still in the trial; she now goes every six months. So far, so good. The amazing thing is that throughout this entire period, she has had no adverse side effects.

Folks, this is a *warrior*! Kris takes one day at a time, enjoying music, scrap booking, and entertaining family and friends—loving every moment with her devoted husband, Chris.

Kris has some sound advice to pass on to our warriors out there:

- Know your body; if something isn't right, insist on further testing.
- Always look at the bright side. She has found a new mission—speaking out about cancer.
- Surround yourself with positive people. Any negativity impedes your healing process.

JILL P.

Biker Babe keeps on kickin' cancer.

This woman gives a new meaning to the word *warrior*. Jill has fought every conceivable battle with cancer and won. Her Blackfoot Indian ancestors are looking down on her with pride.

Jill's journey began in 1977, when she was experiencing such severe pain; she had to have her three-year-old daughter help her up the stairs! A friend suggested she see a doctor. Jill reluctantly agreed, thinking to herself, *Why all the fuss? It's probably only a yeast infection.* Boy was she wrong. After a series of tests, the doctor delivered two powerful blows: she not only had ovarian cancer, but she had only twenty-four hours to live if she didn't have surgery immediately! The doctor informed her that her condition was so severe it could be seen with the naked eye. Surgery, followed by treatment, sent our warrior on the road to recovery—or so she thought.

In 1990 Jill, who is a nurse, noticed a sore on her shoulder, but thought nothing of it. She went to pick up a patient, and the sore literally split open.

She went to the emergency room, and after a series of tests she heard those words everyone dreads—she had cancer, but this time it was basal cell carcinoma, a skin cancer. She underwent skin grafts followed by cauterization, where heat is applied to destroy the cancerous cells.

Jill went on the next fifteen years doing what she loved most: nursing, riding her motorcycle, and driving her Corvette. As you can see, cancer wasn't about to slow this gal down.

In June 2005, Jill discovered a scar on her right eye. Within a couple of weeks the lesion grew and her vision blurred. Due to her history, her doctor referred her to the Wills Eye Hospital in Philadelphia. Travel expenses were provided by the Angel Flight, an organization that helps patients with their transportation problems. After a series of tests, again she was told her cancer was back, only this time in her eye. Again a grim prognosis was given. Jill was told if she didn't have surgery, she would die. Even more devastating, the doctors told her the surgery would save her life, but not her eyesight. Without thinking twice, Jill opted for the surgery. This woman *loves* life!

In spite of the horrific news she was given, all Jill could think about was getting back on her motorcycle.

She had the surgery, which required them to put a radiation plate in her eye. Seven days later she had it removed.

Miraculously, after a month, her vision was 20/20, and no further treatment was needed.

After this Jill continued on her bike, was a New York State Power Lifter for Columbia County, New York, and was a member of ABATE (American Bikers Aim Toward Education). No matter how much cancer was chasing her, she turned around, looked it in the eye, and kicked the daylights out of it.

* I spoke to Jill recently. She told me in August 2009, she began to have vision problems. Glasses weren't doing the trick and she was experiencing sharp pains, so back to the doctors she went. Her retina was detaching to the point it was bulging out. This time it wasn't cancer, but she began getting chemo shots. She went once a month for six months. She then will go back in October to start it again. Her progress will dictate how many treatments she will have. Today Jill substitute teaches kindergarten through twelfth grade, teaches nursing, and *still rides her motorcycle!*

I told you this book will inspire you to fight cancer. Did I lie? Jill is doing all this and is sixty-three years old. This is the definition of a Cancer Kickin' Warrior!

MARK S. DPM

Never, ever give up

I am a cancer warrior. I am writing to share my story with you. Perhaps this story can help some other people. I am fifty-two years old. For the past twenty-five years I have been practicing podiatry in Columbia County I was on staff of the old Greene County Memorial Hospital from 1982 until it closed. Ever since our Catskill hospital closed, I have been an attending physician at Columbia Memorial Hospital. For twenty-five years my family has lived in Catskill. My three daughters are proud graduates of CHS.

I grew up in Far Rockaway, Queens, and I spent the summers of my childhood on the beach, swimming in the ocean, snorkeling, and getting sunburns. I never used sunscreen, and I never wore a hat. But I did have fun.

Let's fast forward to 2003. Just before our twenty-fifth wedding anniversary, my wife noticed a small black dot on the top of my head. A biopsy showed it was melanoma. It was very shallow. The cancer was removed, and a "wide local excision" took off a large part of my scalp. Tests showed that the cancer had not spread. We caught it in time. I was safe, or so we thought.

One morning in October 2006 I coughed up a lot of blood. Tests showed a large tumor in the lower part of my left lung. The melanoma was back. A thoracotomy was performed at St. Peter's Hospital in Albany, and one-half of my left lung was removed. Scans showed that the cancer had not spread beyond the one lung. After the surgery I was evaluated at the University of Pennsylvania and accepted into a clinical trial. They were going to give me an experimental drug designed to stop the melanoma from coming back. Everything looked great. I just needed one more scan before they could start. One problem—the scan showed a tumor in my brain. So it was back to St. Peter's in December 2006 for brain surgery. The tumor was removed, the cancer was gone, and I couldn't walk. My left leg was paralyzed. I went from St. Peter's to Sunnyview Rehabilitation Hospital in Schenectady, and with lots of physical therapy I was soon walking with no problem. Things looked good until a routine scan a few weeks later showed some more brain tumors. It was time for three weeks of radiation therapy. Then the brain quieted down; however, there were more tumors in my lungs and other organs. So in April 2007 I was admitted to Beth Israel Deaconess Medical

Center in Boston for interleukin-2 treatments. One week in, one week home, then another week in. Suffice to say it wasn't pleasant.

Things were quiet until June when some remaining tumors in my brain started to bleed. Back to St. Peter's for another craniotomy. I tolerated that surgery well. Even though there was bleeding and more brain surgery, I came through without a neurological deficit. I could walk, talk, and think without any problems. A few weeks later I had some more radiation to the brain.

Now I'm traveling to Yale in New Haven, Connecticut, every few weeks for a new treatment. The saga continues.

What's amazing is that I feel well (except for needing two naps a day).

What do I hope telling my story will accomplish? Well, first, I want to make sure everyone is aware of the dangers of the sun, even in the winter. You need sun block on the slopes as well as on the beach. Parents protect your children; make sure they always wear sun block and wide-brimmed hats. Don't go to tanning parlors. UV light from the sun or from a spa can kill you. Next, get regular skin exams from a dermatologist or your primary care doctor. And if a mole changes in color, shape, or size, see your doctor right away.

Finally, I want other cancer patients to know that there are wonderfully talented doctors, nurses, and other health-care providers out there who can help you get through this.

Don't despair. There are great breakthroughs coming every day. The treatment that appears to be helping me now wasn't even around a few years ago. Don't be afraid to ask questions. It's your body.

* Now, people, hold onto your seats. This is now 2010; I want you to take a peek at my latest letter from Dr. S.

When I wrote to you three years ago, I said that I wasn't a statistic and even though the life expectancy of someone with stage 4 melanoma was less than one year, I knew that some people survived, so why wouldn't it be me. My perseverance has paid off. Thanks to a new drug called Ipilimumab, which I first received on Halloween in 2007, I am now cancer free. My oncologist told me the great news two months ago. Ipilimumab doesn't kill cancer; it altered my immune system so that my body could find and destroy the melanoma cells. This drug is still considered experimental, but it looks like the FDA may approve it this year. You may have seen news reports about "Ipi" earlier this month. It is the first drug that has been shown to extend the lives of some stage 4 melanoma patients. The treatment isn't pleasant, and it doesn't work on everybody, but it saved my life.

My journey since I was first diagnosed with advanced melanoma in 2006 has been long and frightening. I have had four major surgeries, radiation treatments, other cancer drugs, and many emergency hospital admissions when things looked very bad. I have received treatment in five different cancer centers in four different states. I can now say that I am a cancer survivor.

I did not travel down this road alone. I wrote to you about my family three years ago. My wife and three daughters have all supported me with strength I did not know they had. They were there for every surgery, every stay in the ICU, and every hospital admission. They saw me lose forty pounds and all my hair. They helped carry me and dress me when I was too weak to do it myself. They supported each other during the tough times, and they never failed to let me know how much they loved me. During this journey my eldest daughter gave birth to my first grandchild, Tyler.

My wife is my hero. She was always there with me, every single day, and has driven over a thousand miles taking me to and from doctor appointments.

When I wrote my reflections on cancer, which you were kind enough to publish in 2007, I did not expect to be here three years later. Thanks to cancer researchers, fantastic doctors, a wonderful family, and a health insurance company (CDPHP) that was willing to pay for tests and treatments in all these different out-of-area hospitals, I am alive today.

Cancer patients *must* be their own advocates. Make sure you are receiving treatment at a center that specializes in your particular type of cancer. Never hesitate to get a second or third opinion. Understand all your options, and ask questions. No matter what the odds, if some people with your diagnosis have survived, you may be a survivor too.

* For all of you, who think about giving up, think again!

THE SOLDIERS

We praise our warriors for their courage and strength In the battle against cancer. But as powerful as we are, we couldn't go against the force of cancer, without the people that stand beside us, with us, and for us. In some cases they fight when we can't. They speak when we can't. In other words, they are our soldiers. These are just a few of the soldiers that have crossed our paths. We know their compassion. We marvel at the strength and tenacity they exhibit while joining forces with us in the fight against this enemy.

Patrick DiPaolo, MD

Dr. Patrick DiPaolo is a doctor of hematology and oncology who practices in Montclair, New Jersey. He has been in practice for twenty years. DiPaolo received his degree in medicine from Università Degli Studi di Roma la Sapienza (Facoltà l) in Italy.

Dr. DiPaolo is both a member of and physician for the New Jersey State Law Enforcement Officers Association. He received the Patients' Choice Award in 2008, 2009, and 2010. In the November 2007 issue of *New Jersey*, he was listed among the 573 top doctors and 56 specialists. Dr. DiPaolo was also the recipient of the Squibb Humanitarian Award for Humanistic Qualities. It's little wonder that his patients give him a four-star rating, and I can see why.

Dr. Patrick DiPaolo is one of the reasons I'm here today. I am not just referring to his expertise in the fields of oncology and hematology; but more important, the encouragement and support he gave me to fight cancer. In 2001, I walked into his office asking him how long I had to live. To this day I remember his response: "If you do what I say, I can only guarantee you'll live to be ninety. After that, I can't guarantee anything."

Folks, at the time the only thing I knew about cancer was that if you had it—you die! Hearing his words gave me the kick I needed to proceed with my treatments.

He takes his time with every patient, and more important, he explains it in the simplest terms. He always greets me with a smile, and after hearing one of his corny jokes, I leave with a smile. He never gives up on his patients.

To this day, I take the long drive to his office, because I trust him with my life. We all know in battling any life-threatening illness, having a doctor you can trust is the most important thing to your recovery.

Dr. DiPaolo, you are my doctor; but more important, you are my friend.

Sabrina Mosseau, BSRN, OCN

Sabrina has been an oncology nurse for over twelve years. Her entire career has been spent at Northeast Health, as an inpatient oncology nurse, as an oncology clinical nurse specialist, and her current role as the Administrative Director of Medical Oncology and Women's Health for Samaritan Hospital. In her own words, "I truly love my job role and the responsibilities to make sure quality and service are number one priorities. The care of people living with cancer is my passion … I believe sincerely that we have a responsibility to continue to challenge the health-care system and exceed expectations in providing quality, comprehensive patient-centered care. We need to realize that treatment is not only about surgery, radiation, and chemotherapy, but about pushing the envelope to make sure that the people we care for have access to patient navigators and integrative wellness: nutritional counseling, psychosocial support, massage, healing touch, Reiki, and whatever modality does not cause harm but can certainly make people live better with their disease.

"These are my passion points."

So often we praise our physician, technologies and researchers; that we sometimes forget the very people who work the closest with us—our nurses. When we open our eyes for the first time after surgery, they are usually the first ones we see—the first ones to comfort us. Sabrina's own words paint a picture for us that show the strength, compassion, and dedication they have to have to deal with this disease on a daily basis.

Let us not forget these soldiers that are on the forefront.

BENITA ZAHN

Folks, first I want to tell you about the extensive background of a woman I highly admire. Benita Zahn co-anchors NewsChannel 13 Live at 5 and 6. In her position of health reporter, she is on the forefront of any issues surrounding medical breakthroughs, nutrition, aging, health trends—she does it all. If it's new or upcoming, Benita knows about it. And what she knows you'll know. In addition to this she co-produces and hosts *Health Link*, which is aired on WMHT on Thursday.

Her accomplishments speak for themselves. Her list of awards includes being named one of the 100 Women of the Century by the Albany-Colonie Regional Chamber of Commerce; three-time Emmy nominee; a gold medal in the 1995 New York Festivals International Television competition for "Baby Your Baby"; the Distinguished Communicator Award from American Women in Radio and Television; 1997 YMCA Citizen of the Year; the New York State Health Education Week Award; and media awards from the American Cancer

Society, the American Lung Association, and the American Heart Association.

She is the community member for the St. Peter's Hospital Ethics Board and honorary chair for the Susan G. Komen Breast Cancer Run. In 2009, Benita received her master's degree in bioethics at Albany Medical College. Though she is a beautiful woman, she is not just a pretty face

In spite of all of these accomplishments, I admire her for something much more: her compassion, commitment, and love she gives to people.

It seemed like when I participated in any cancer walk, fund-raiser, or program, Benita was there. I have appeared on her shows, and I can tell you the emotions that pour through her eyes when interviewing a cancer survivor are real. She is a tireless crusader and motivator. Sometimes I think the only words in her vocabulary are, "What can I do for you? What do you need? Remember, I'm here."

Benita, I thank you for being our voice.

Harvey Zimbler, MD

You read the amazing story about my personal hero and friend, Bootie Fenoff; now read her story praising the remarkable doctor who continues to be her knight in shining armor.

Dr. Harvey Zimbler specializes in internal medicine, oncology, and hematology. His expertise lies in the fields of adult T-cell leukemia-lymphoma, cancer prevention, and epidemiology. He has been practicing for over thirty-five years.

Bootie says she finds it hard to put into words, what a great doctor he is. He is compassionate, knowledgeable, passionate, and friendly, and he has a memory that doesn't quit. He has been her doctor for eighteen years; and she trusts him immensely. Bootie has a special note for Dr. Zimbler: "Please don't ever retire."

KATIE V.

Through a daughter's eyes

On a cool fall Sunday afternoon, I found myself in a familiar place: Yankee Stadium. It was September 19, 2004, and my mom and I were at our usual Sunday hangout. Except this time it was under different circumstances. We were in the shady handicap seats in the main level watching the Yankees pummel Pedro Martinez and the Boston Red Sox. However, this was not our normal vantage point. Our Sunday season tickets in a tier box were in the sun, a place not conducive for someone undergoing chemotherapy. My mom had been diagnosed with stage 2 breast cancer in June of that year. While we were thrilled at what was going on in the game, my mom's hair was beginning to fall out very quickly. It was a scary sight for me to see the physical manifestation of the treatments.

The baseball was a welcomed distraction from the harsh realities of the cancer. Since my first game at Yankee Stadium as a six-year-old in 1994, I was hooked. As a former fast-pitch softball pitcher, my mom taught me a love for the games of baseball and softball. It was this devotion to the sport and the love of the Yankees that helped us get through a difficult time. We had tickets to every Sunday game that season and did not miss one, even through the surgery in July and chemotherapy treatments in the fall. Even though my mom was faced with an incredibly challenging situation, she was always in great spirits and taught me a great deal about how to handle life's hardships. After experiencing how cancer affected my mom, I became involved in the Penn State Dance Marathon, which raises money ($7.48 million as a school just this year) to cure childhood cancer. That experience will culminate this fall when I will be a Thon chair for the Kinesiology Club at Penn State. I believe it is necessary to help those that are going through the same experiences that you have gone through.

From the initial conversation of breaking the news about my mom's cancer to the excitement when the doctors declared her cancer free, the battle with cancer is a roller-coaster ride no one wants to be on. However, once the ride is over, it stays with us forever. Whether taking part in fund-raisers or simply wearing a pink ribbon, we hold the memory of what we have been through and the hope for those that will face it in the future and, eventually finding a cure. Perhaps nothing exemplifies our devotion to the Yankees more than my mom and I sitting glued to the TV the night before her surgery on July 1, 2004, as Derek Jeter dove into the stands during that never-ending game. It was baseball that helped us through then, and continues to be the best distraction of them all.

* Katie, who also was a member of the Honor Society, has since graduated. She is looking into graduate school to pursue her career as a physician's assistant.

GREENE COUNTY WOMEN'S LEAGUE CANCER PATIENT AID

As a cancer survivor, I know firsthand the changes your mind goes through when you're diagnosed with cancer. In addition to dealing with the medical decisions, you worry about cost, wondering how much your insurance will pay. I know of a woman diagnosed with breast cancer, who had insurance, but just the amount of the co-pay and medicine proved to be a hardship. Unfortunately, during this time of rising fuel and food prices, this is a story I hear over and over again. Greene County, New York, is very fortunate to have an organization that tries to assist with the costs.

The Greene County Women's League Cancer Patient Aid is a not-for-profit organization that is dedicated to assisting people in Greene County who have had the misfortune of being diagnosed with cancer. The organization was started about thirty-five years ago by a group of women from the Catskill area. Even though these women were well insured, they worried about the person who wasn't as fortunate. What would they do if they were hit with a diagnosis of cancer? That was the beginning of the Greene County Women's League Cancer Patient Aid.

They raise monies through fund-raisers and through the generosity of people and businesses in Greene County. The league assists with expenses incurred with the diagnosis and treatment of cancer. They help pay for doctor bills, pharmacy expenses, hospital costs, wigs, breast prostheses, transportation for treatment, etc. As stated in their bylaws, all information pertaining to their clients must be held in the strictest of confidence. They do not, however, pay for Medicaid patients, as Social Services pays for all of the patient's medical expenses. At the present time, the Greene County Women's League will pay up to $1,500 per patient. Anything over and above that amount must be approved by the officers and board of directors and then brought to the membership for a majority vote.

I am proud to say that I joined this organization because I was so impressed by their dedication and tireless work they do for cancer patients.

In these trying times, it is so wonderful to know there are people like the Greene County Women's League who devote their time and energy, while pouring their heart and soul, into helping people struggling with cancer.

* Greene County is a rural area. There are no buses, so it can be costly and difficult for a person to travel thirty-five miles to the main hospitals in Albany.

HOPE NEMIROFF

People, so often when we are diagnosed with a serious illness, we want to forget about it, put it behind us after treatment. Cancer is so traumatic; believe me, I can understand why someone would think like this. But then you have the survivors—the soldiers, if you will—that remember those feelings and want to reach out and touch another human being experiencing those feelings. This is what Hope Nemiroff is all about. I know her personally and can tell you that her selflessness and compassion, coupled with a yearning for more information about this disease, turned an idea into a growing organization. When you read Hope's story, you will see why I have such love and respect for this woman.

Hope Nemiroff was diagnosed with breast cancer in 1994. Facing a life-threatening illness, she decided to learn everything she could about the disease so that she could make the best choices for her own medical care. It is during this time that Hope came to understand that her experience was also the experience of hundreds of thousands of women each year.

She discovered that not all physicians in the rapidly growing field of breast cancer treatment were practicing according to a consistent set of guidelines, that patients were overwhelmed and frightened and often had neither the experiences nor the resources to seek good care, much less receive the support that would sustain them, and that in the explosion of new treatment modalities (both traditional and complementary) very few physicians or patients understood their options.

She founded Breast Cancer Options in 2000. As executive director, she oversees and organizes support, education, and advocacy programs for Breast Cancer Options and has expanded them into a six-county area to make sure that all patients have the information and support they need to make informed medical decisions.

She spearheaded a research project with Sheldon M. Feldman, MD, to study the pesticide levels in body fat of breast cancer patients and designed the research questionnaire for the project, which was funded by national foundations. She is coauthor of "DDT May Be a Contaminant in Green Tea from China," with Devra Davis, PhD, and Sheldon M. Feldman, MD. She was cited for contributing background materials for "Life's Delicate Balance: Causes and Prevention of Breast Cancer," by Janette D. Sherman, MD. Hope provided material for the Vassar College interactive CD-ROM, "Environmental Risks and Breast Cancer" and developed a Healthy Lifestyle Calendar with practical information on how to minimize environmental exposures for the consumer. Thirty thousand of these calendars have been distributed, and it has been used as a teaching tool by other organizations and in schools. She attends environmental conferences, organizes environmental programs, and works to focus attention on the environmental risks we all face on a daily basis.

Hope is a founding board member of the New York State Breast Cancer Network, the only statewide network of community-based breast cancer organizations in the country.

She has served as a consumer advocate reviewer for the New York State Health Research Science Board Breast Cancer Funding Review Committee for breast cancer studies.

She wrote and compiled the *Breast Cancer Resource Guide*, which is distributed throughout the Hudson Valley, and an *Ovarian Cancer Resource Guide* for the Linda Young Ovarian Cancer Support Program at Benedictine Hospital, Kingston, New York.

She produces a yearly integrative medicine conference that has nationwide attendance and exposure.

Breast Cancer Options offers the following services: Companion Advocates, Camp LightHeart, Acupuncture Clinics, BCO News, Annual Complementary Medicine Conference, Breast Cancer Resource Guide, Referrals for Financial and Legal Problems, Discount Vitamin Club, Lend-A-Helping-Hand, Peer to Peer Mentoring, and Healthy Lifestyles Calendar.

LESLEY R. RAFES

I have four cousins and a sister-in-law, all survivors, all within the past fifteen years so I have been a part of their stories and struggles through it all. One day I was reading a magazine, and I saw an ad to be part of the cure for breast cancer by participating in a three-day sixty-mile walk in New York City … not knowing anything about it, I signed up to be on the motorcycle safety crew and figured I'd volunteer my time, raise a little money, and do my good deed for the weekend. *Well …* let me tell you something, there is nothing like cheering on six thousand walkers through the streets of New York City for three days and sixty miles. The amazing courage, strength, and beauty that I saw in these women absolutely blew me away! I guided them through the five boroughs, kept them safe along the busy streets, and urged them on when they thought they couldn't take another step but what they did for me was beyond words. These women (and men)—some survivors, some walking for lost loved ones, and some walking for every grandmother, mother, and daughter—showed me that the power of one step is as strong as the power of every dollar raised. Here I was, riding my motorcycle all over the city, smiling, laughing, cheering on the walkers   my bike covered with pink ribbons, a pink seat cover, and pink plush boobies on the windshield, and these walkers were thanking *me* for being there! They were tired, dirty, blistered, and sore, yet they were thanking me for volunteering for the event.

When day 3 arrived and it was getting close to the last mile all of the bikers on the moto-safety crew got behind the very last of the walkers   As they crossed the finish line to cheers and yells from friends and family, we followed behind, flashing our lights, blowing the horns, and feeling the love from everyone involved in this event! After parking the bikes and listening to the closing remarks, I was overwhelmed with emotion. I cried buckets   I cried for every one of those six thousand walkers. I cried for all of their pain and for their struggle to survive. For every walker I hugged and said, "Congratulations. I'm so proud of you" one said they couldn't have done it without the moto-safety crew keeping them safe and supporting them through it all … We were the first ones out on the route every morning and the last ones in every night! It was the most rewarding, spiritually satisfying, exhausting, blissful weekend of my life!

That was nine years ago   I haven't missed an event since! The three-day walk in New York became the Avon Breast Cancer 2-day Walk a few years ago, and the moto-safety is one of the most popular of all the volunteer crews   how can we not be   we love and protect our walkers every minute of every mile!

The funniest thing about my motorcycle ... the "pink" stays on all year round! I ride my bike to work with all the pink breast cancer ribbons on it. No matter what motorcycle event I participate in, someone usually thanks me for wearing the ribbons and then shares their story with me. Every year immediately after the walk, with my voice hoarse from cheering, my body tired from riding, my eyes wet with tears, and my heart so full of love it wants to burst, I sign up to do it again!

Looking forward to October 2010 in New York City! *Moto crew rocks!*

Words of Wisdom

Warriors, I want to pass along some words of wisdom I've learned through my Cancer Kickin' Journey.

- Don't let anyone determine when you are going to die. Think of anyone you know (young or old)—do you know how long they have to live? Remember, cancer just means you have something with a name to it, period! No life is guaranteed.

- Don't obsess or even look at statistics. You don't know how they were compiled. They may include people who never sought treatment for their cancer. Everyone is different.

- Chemotherapy can be debilitating, but so can death. Make your own decision whether to get it or not. Just remember, whatever you decide, fight like hell and give it all you've got.

- No matter what medical process you chose while going through cancer (holistic or pharmaceutical), don't bad-mouth another person's choice. Remember, if we all knew the right cures for cancer, we all would be healed and cancer would be a thing of the past.

+ Stay away from negativity. Examine your so-called friends. Look at them more closely. If they are injecting poison or negativity—get rid of them.

+ Do not make any life-changing decisions while going through treatment. Healing and recuperating should be the only thing on your mind.

+ Know your body. If something is not right, have it checked out.

+ Do not let your doctor talk you out of getting a test done. If he isn't fixing the problem—*change doctors, get more tests.* Remember, the idea is to catch it *before* it spreads.

+ Continue seeing an oncologist even after treatment, no matter how many years have gone by. Remember, cancer is a sneaky culprit.

+ If your pharmaceutical drugs are too costly, contact the drug company directly. A lot of them have special programs. Some include free drugs.

+ If you need medication immediately and can't afford it, ask your doctor for those samples that the pharmaceutical companies give them to push their products.

+ Keep those good looks. You do not have to wear

the "**cancer mask.**" This is not a vanity issue; it's a mental health issue.

+ *Above all, don't be afraid of cancer; be afraid if you don't do anything about it!*

REMEMBER, YOU ARE NOT JUST A SURVIVOR BUT A CANCER KICKIN' WARRIOR!

POEM

This is a poem I wrote that expresses how I felt when I was diagnosed with breast cancer.

I'll Cry Tomorrow

By Inez Dickens

Another day has come, but I miss the night
Because I don't have to think, about what's right

But this thing is growing, so do I dare say
If I don't think about it, it will go away

I haven't cried, since given the news
No time to cry, there's so much to choose

If they take a small section, it may come back
If I go with the chemo, I'll be wearing a hat

If I choose radiation, do I want the burn?
Or do I remove it completely, with no return?

So today is for decisions, my time is borrowed
I've made up my mind, I'll cry tomorrow

And when and where I cry, don't pity me
'Cause these tears will bring, the fight in me

They'll be tears of strength, no tears of sorrow
But it won't be today, 'cause I'll cry tomorrow!

NOW, ARE YOU A CANCER KICKIN' WARRIOR?

LaVergne, TN USA
29 September 2010
198988LV00003B/1/P